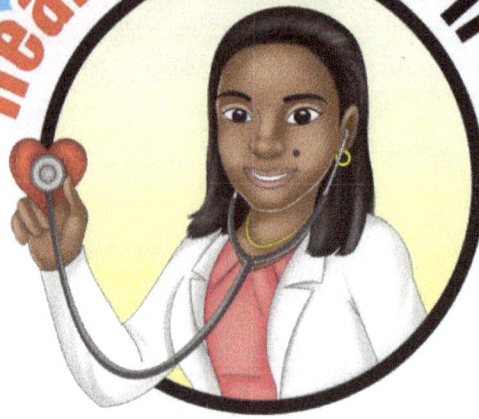

# THIS BOOK BELONGS TO

_____

_____

_____

# HEALTH, HYGIENE AND ANATOMY

## ACTIVITY AND COLORING HANDBOOK FOR KIDS

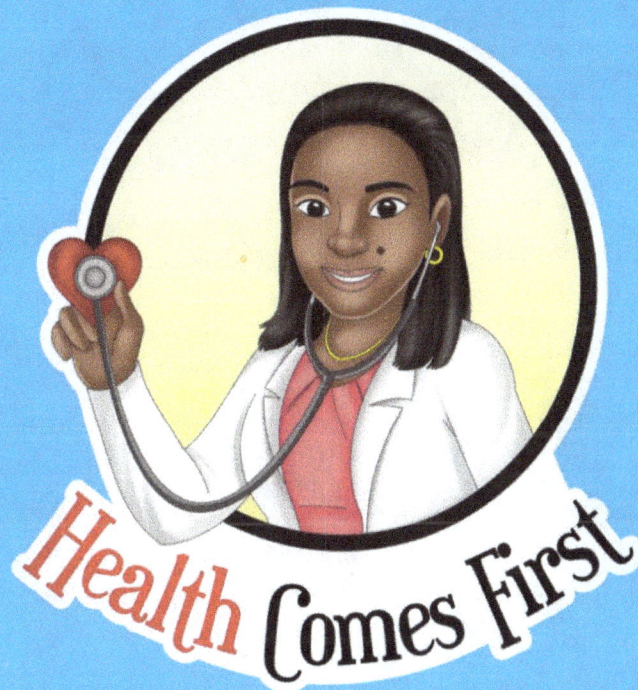

Health Comes First

Written by: T. C. Pask & Dr. A. Francis

# MAZE

Help the sick kids find Doctor Francis

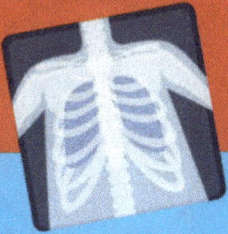

# HUMAN BODY

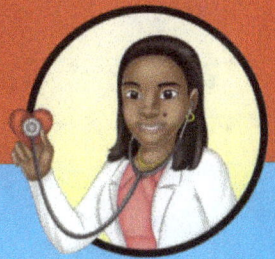

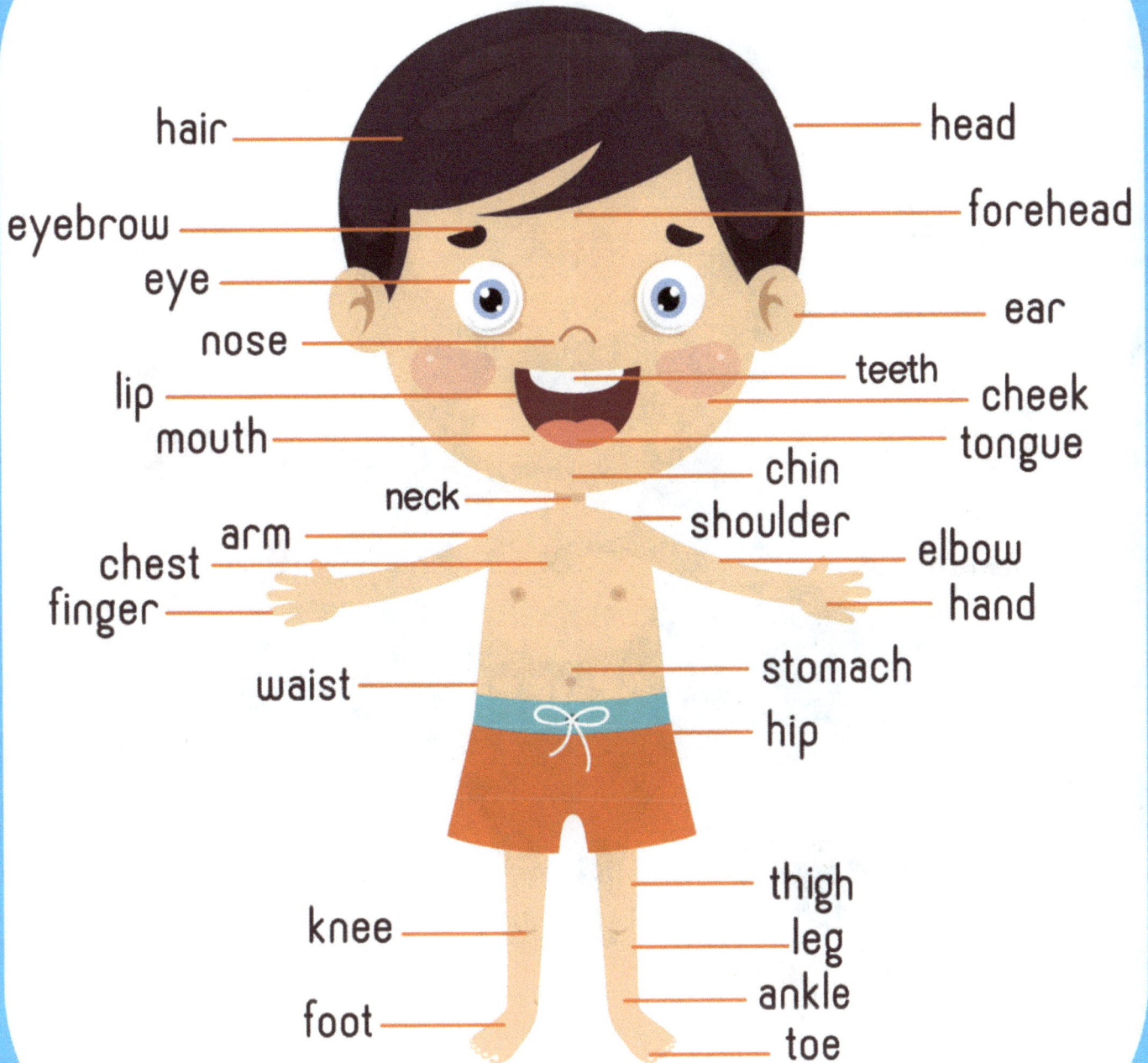

hair

head

forehead

eyebrow

eye

ear

nose

teeth

cheek

lip

mouth

tongue

chin

neck

shoulder

arm

elbow

chest

finger

hand

waist

stomach

hip

thigh

knee

leg

ankle

foot

toe

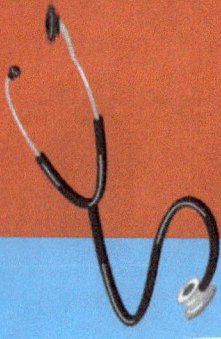
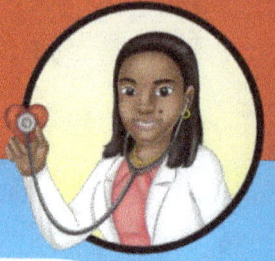

# 5 SENSES

**TOUCH**

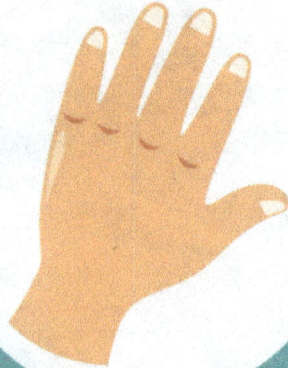

**SMELL**

**TASTE**

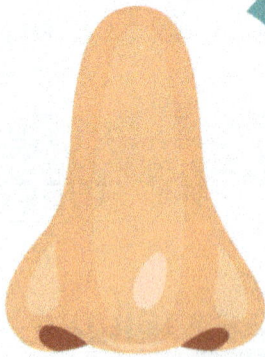

## 5 SENSES

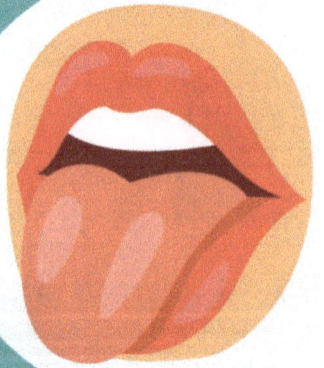

**SIGHT**

**HEARING**

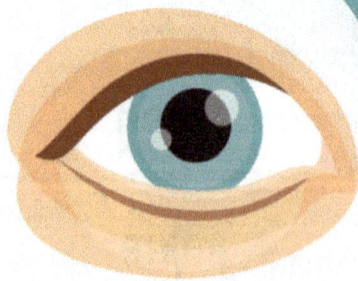
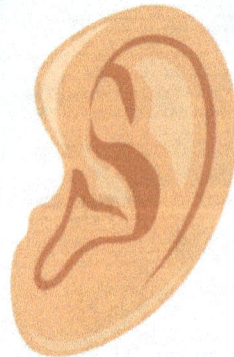

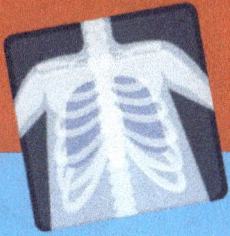

# HUMAN BODY

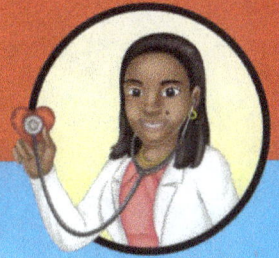

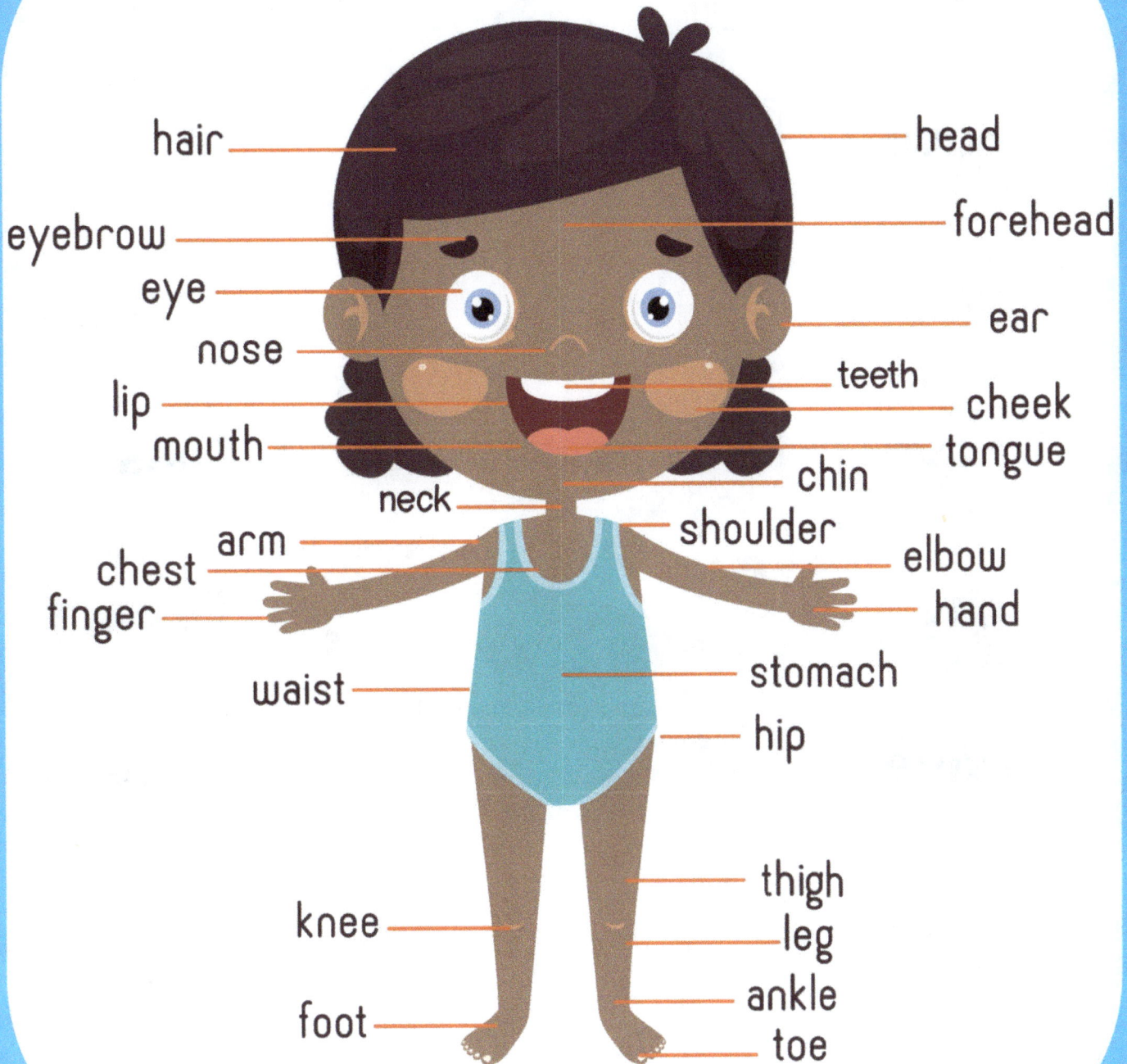

hair

head

forehead

eyebrow

eye

ear

nose

teeth

cheek

lip

tongue

mouth

chin

neck

shoulder

arm

elbow

chest

hand

finger

waist

stomach

hip

thigh

knee

leg

ankle

foot

toe

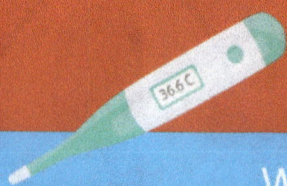

# BODY PARTS

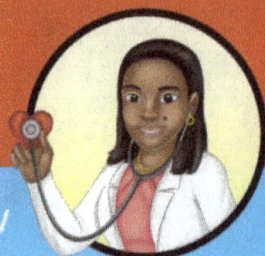

Write the correct number in each box below

I have ☐ 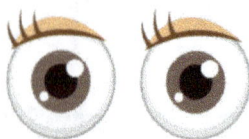 Eyes

I have ☐ 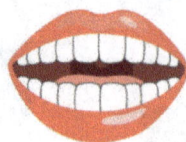 Mouth

I have ☐ 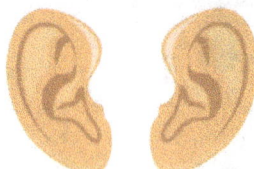 Ears

I have ☐ 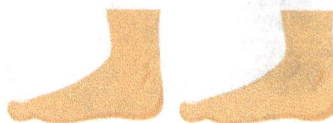 Toes

I have ☐ 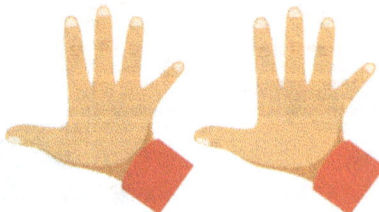 Fingers

I have ☐ Nose

I have ☐ 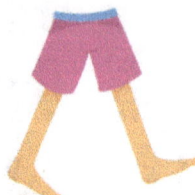 Legs

I have ☐ 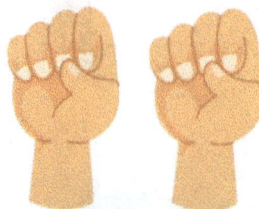 Hands

# HUMAN BODY

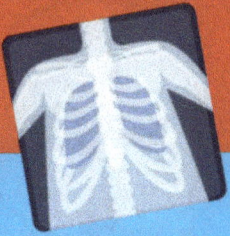
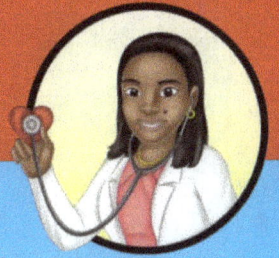

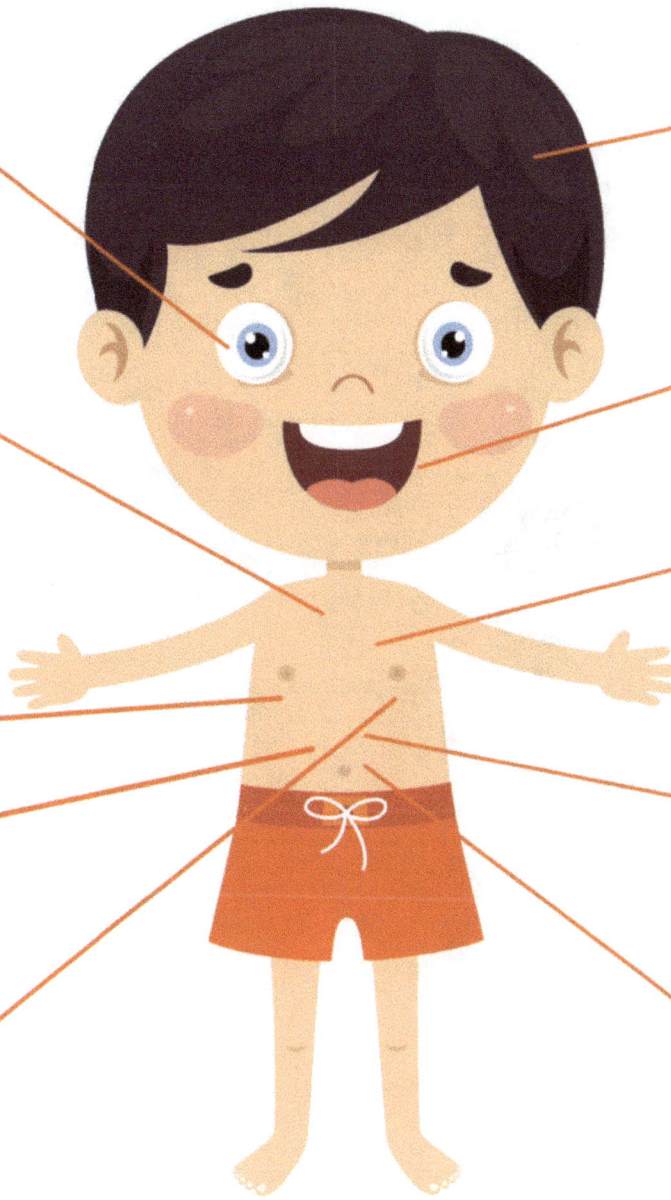

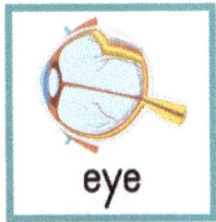
eye

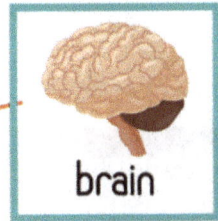
brain

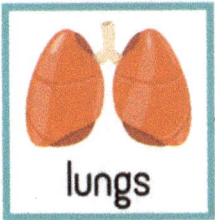
lungs

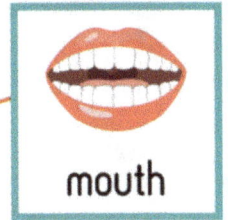
mouth

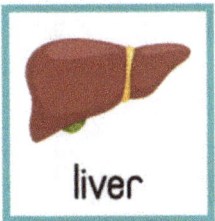
liver

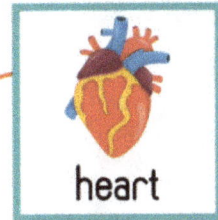
heart

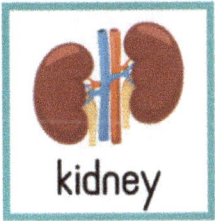
kidney

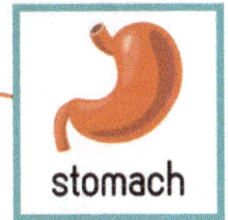
stomach

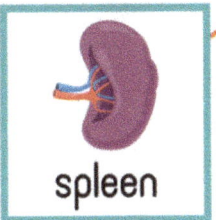
spleen

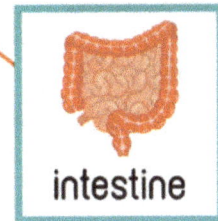
intestine

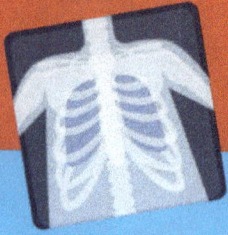

# HUMAN BODY SYSTEMS

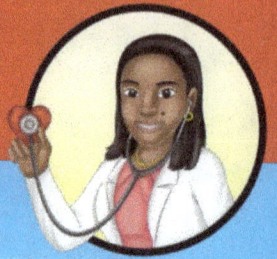

| SKELETAL | CIRCULATORY | NERVOUS | DIGESTIVE |
|---|---|---|---|

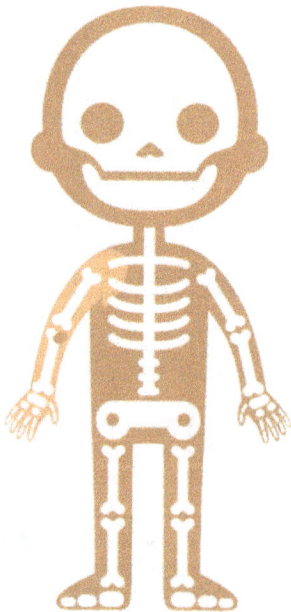 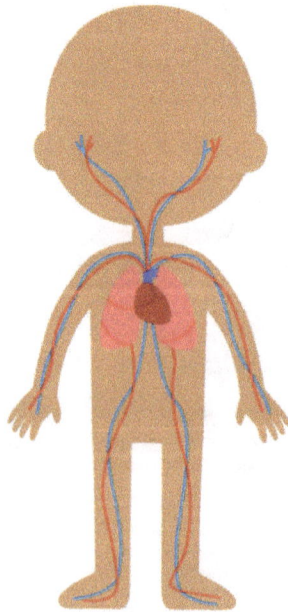 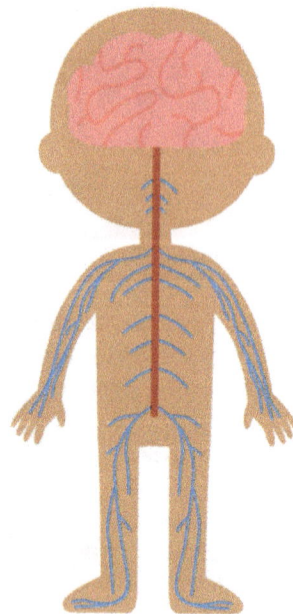 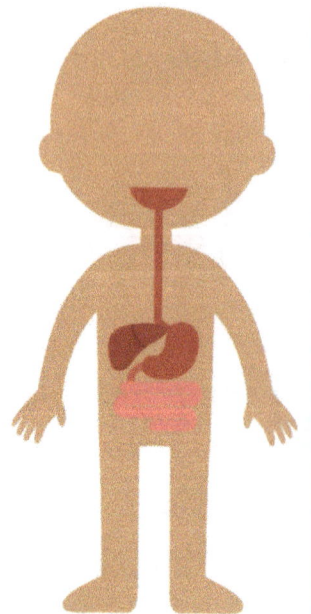

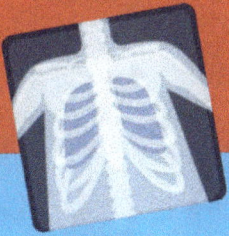

# HUMAN BODY

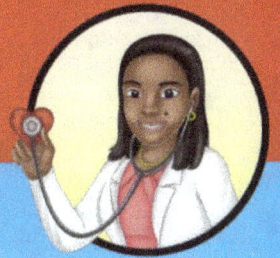

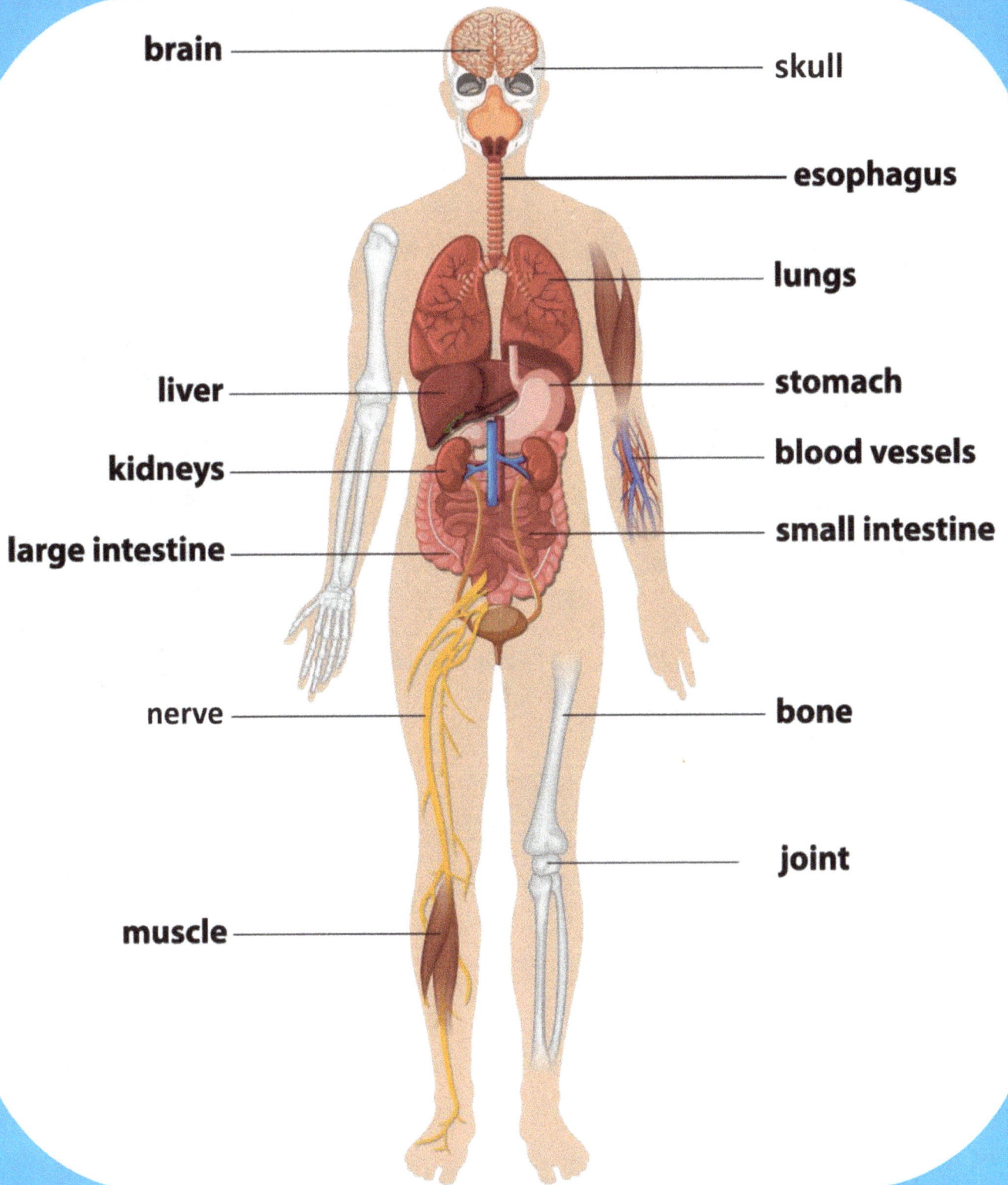

brain

skull

esophagus

lungs

liver

stomach

kidneys

blood vessels

large intestine

small intestine

nerve

bone

joint

muscle

# MATCHING

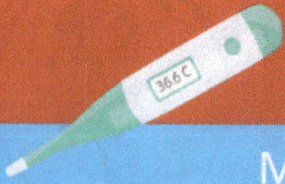

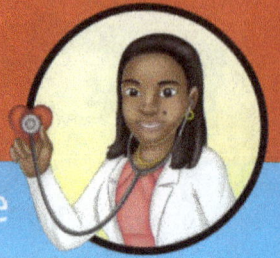

Match each sense with the correct picture

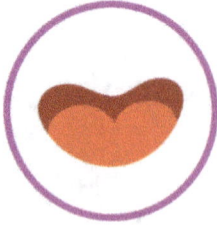

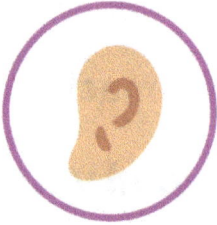

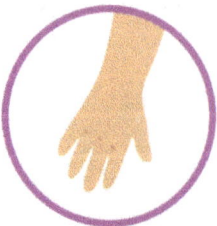

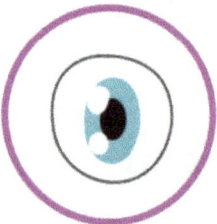

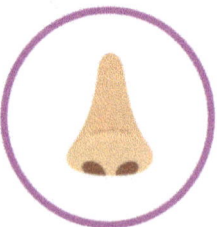

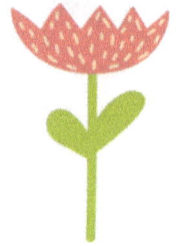

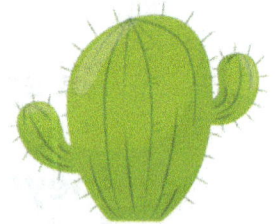

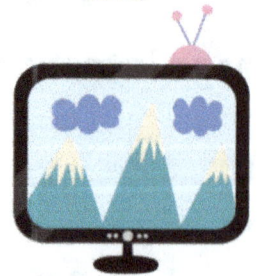

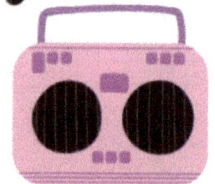

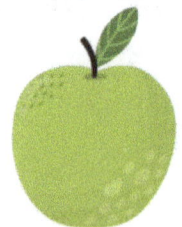

# CROSSWORDS

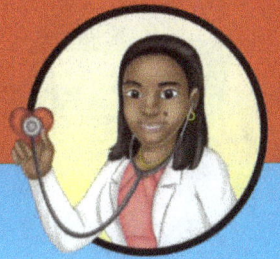

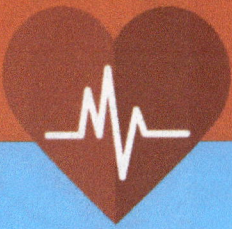

## Fill the boxes with the name of each fruit

1 Strawberry, 4 Grapefruit, 5 Raspberry, 7 Pear
2 Kiwi Fruit, 3 Mango, 6 Apple, 8 Plum, 9 Blueberry, 10 Orange

# HUMAN BODY

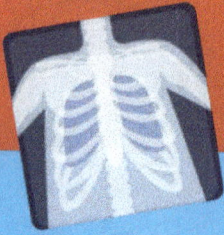
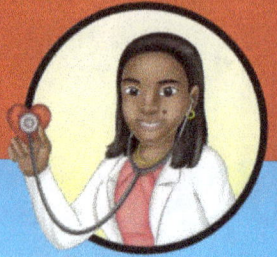

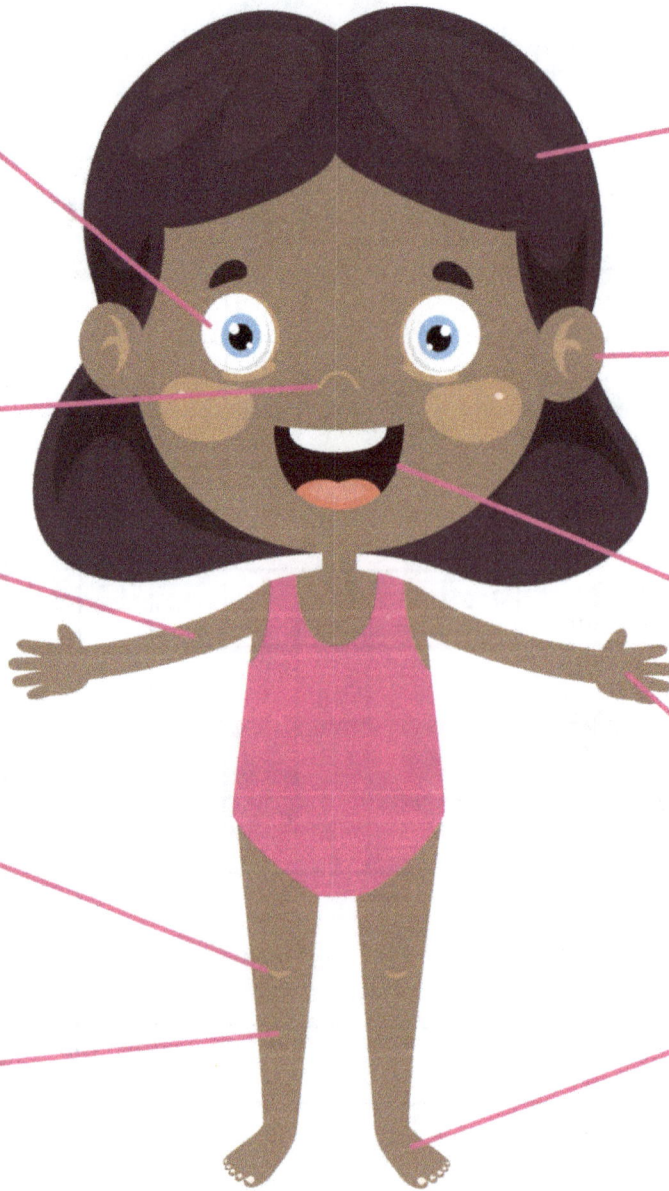

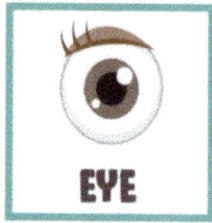
**EYE**

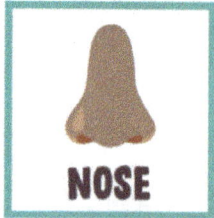
**NOSE**

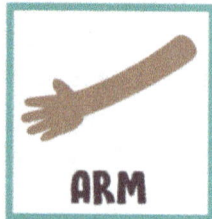
**ARM**

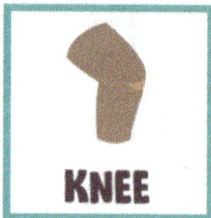
**KNEE**

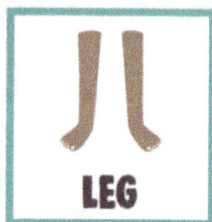
**LEG**

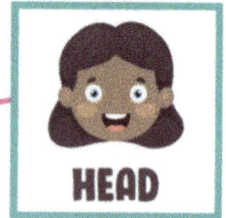
**HEAD**

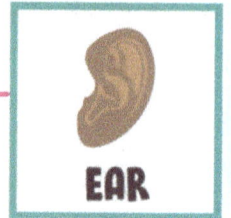
**EAR**

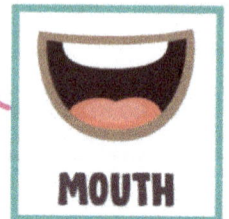
**MOUTH**

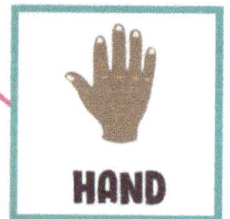
**HAND**

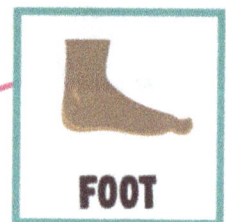
**FOOT**

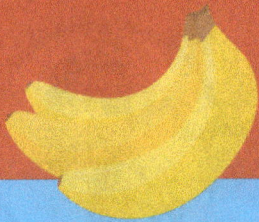

# HUMAN BODY

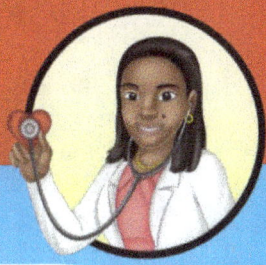

I eat balanced meals

I eat from all the food groups.

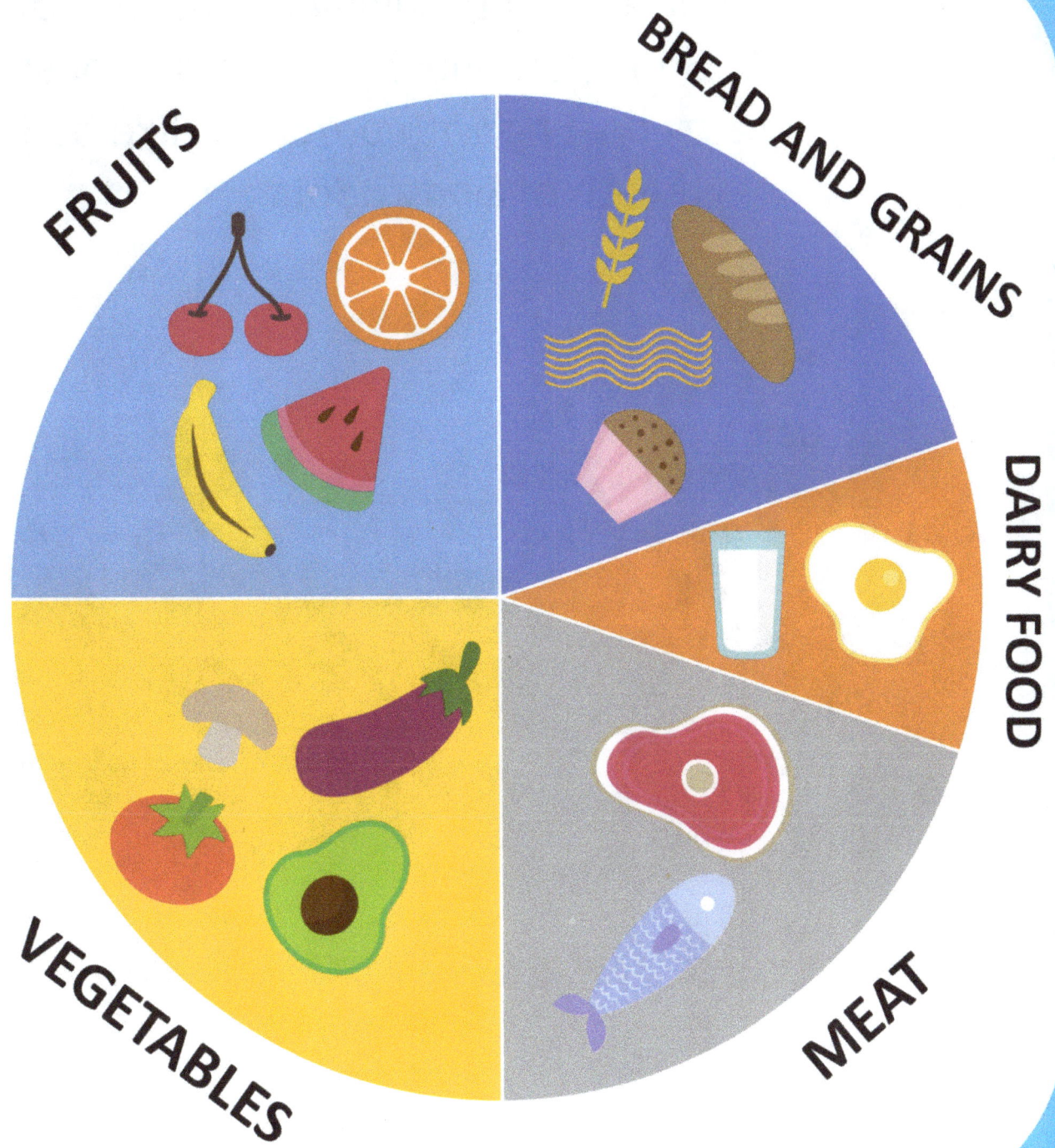

FRUITS

BREAD AND GRAINS

DAIRY FOOD

MEAT

VEGETABLES

# KEEP YOUR BODY CLEAN

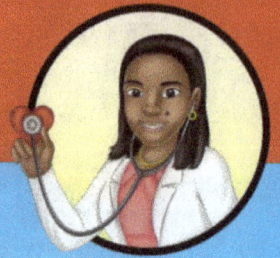

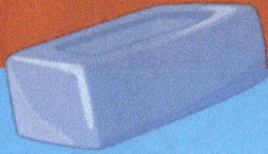

Keep your bodies clean by killing germs to avoid getting sick. Good personal hygiene also boosts confidence by dealing with problems like bad breath or body odour.

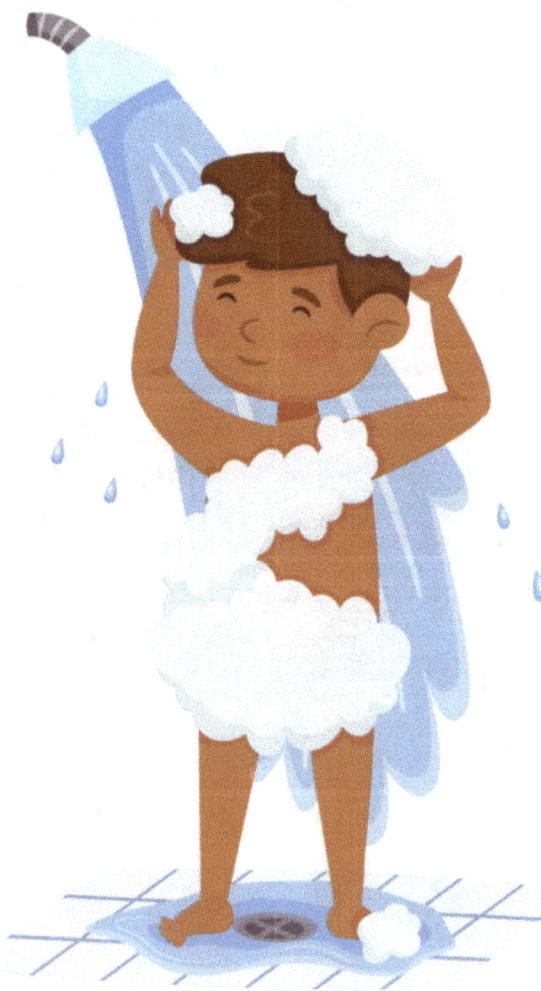

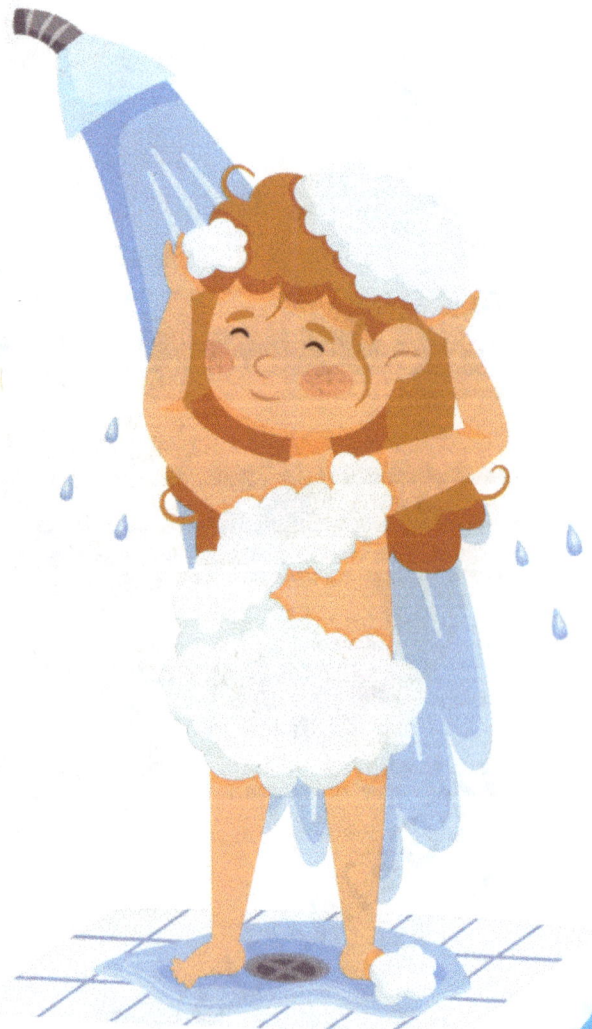

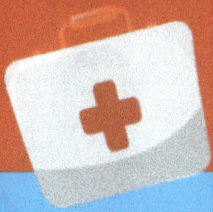

# CONNECTING DOTS

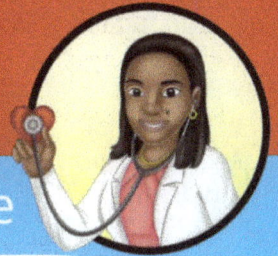

Connect the dots and color the picture

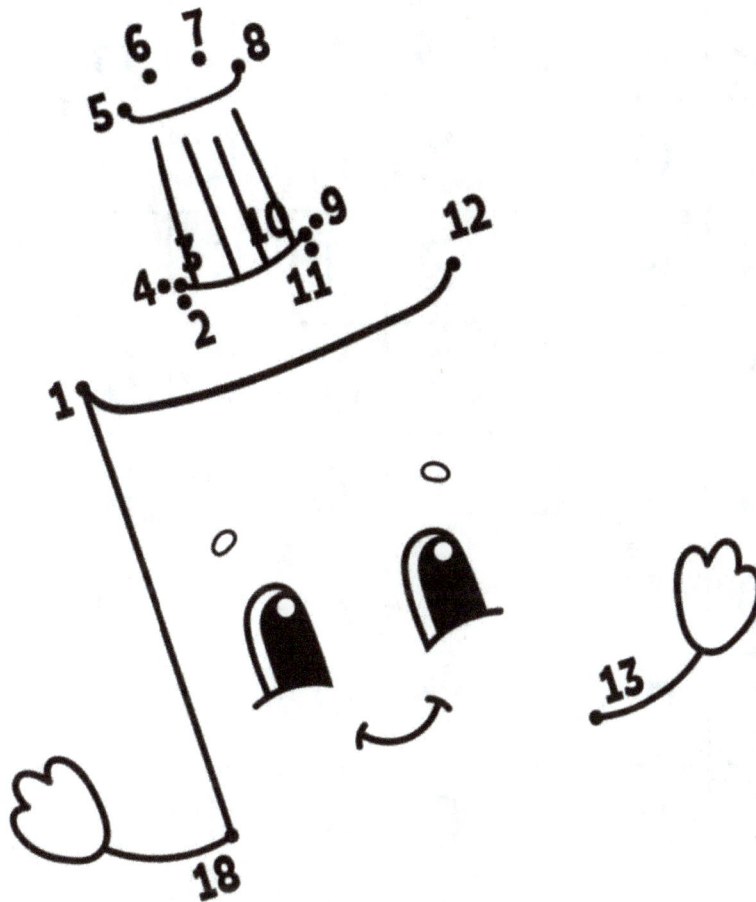

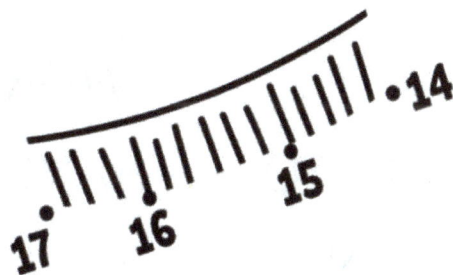

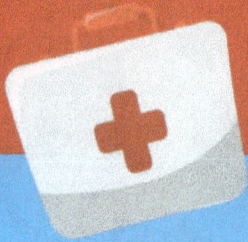

# WORD SEARCH

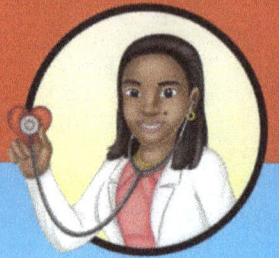

Find the hidden words

| G | T | A | T | O | R | S | H | J | W |
| H | K | O | B | X | H | E | A | D | L |
| M | H | N | E | Z | T | S | L | K | F |
| E | A | R | T | S | Y | E | B | C | I |
| W | N | X | L | I | G | H | K | V | N |
| Q | D | A | F | S | A | C | N | L | G |
| F | E | R | U | V | H | O | E | A | E |
| O | J | M | Y | E | A | Y | E | S | R |
| O | A | G | S | N | G | U | B | V | S |
| T | S | T | O | M | A | C | H | B | K |

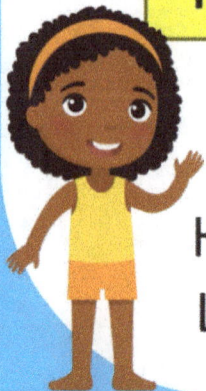

## WORDS

HEAD – TOES – HAND – FOOT – FINGERS

LEG – KNEE – STOMACH – ARM – CHEST

# GUESS THE NAME

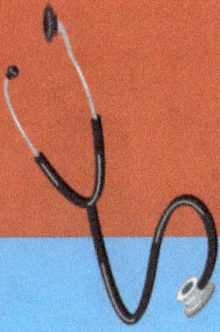

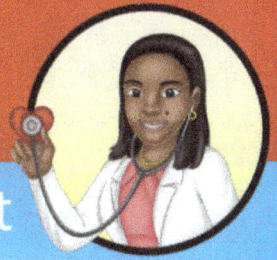

## Write the name of each body part

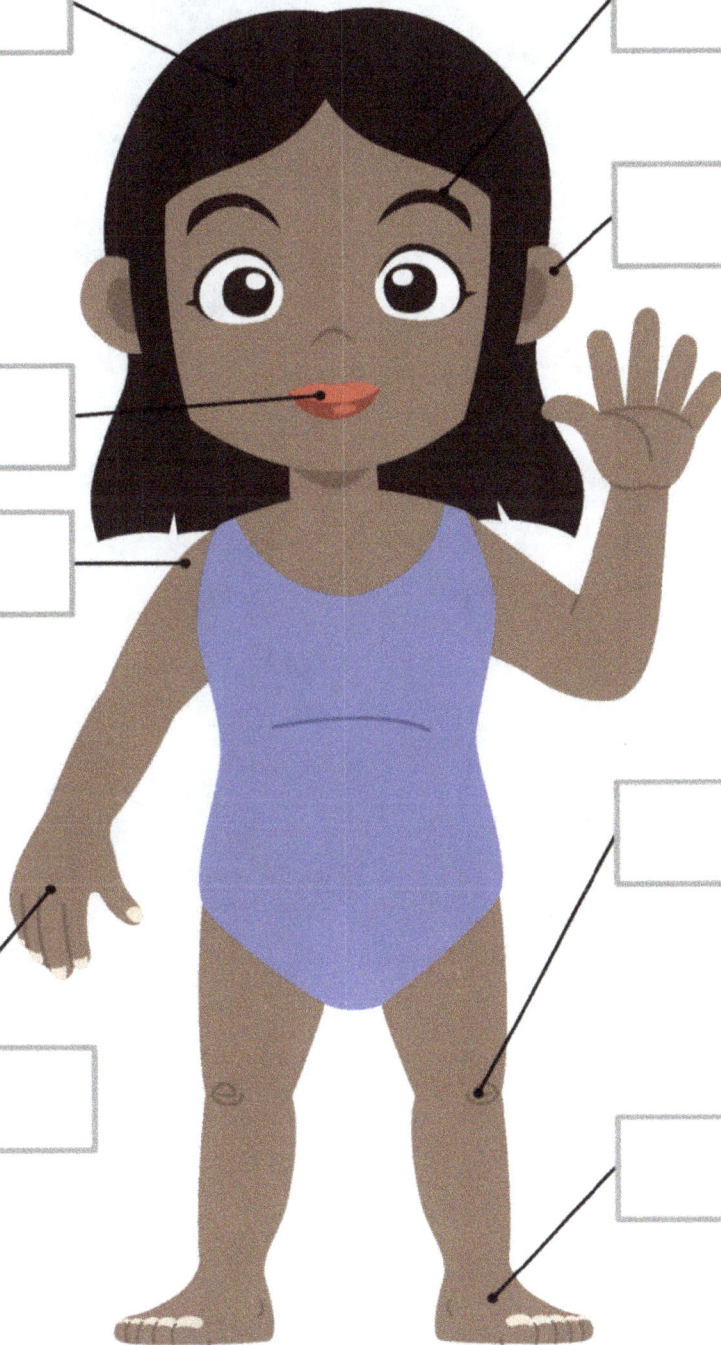

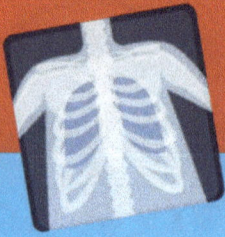

# HUMAN BODY

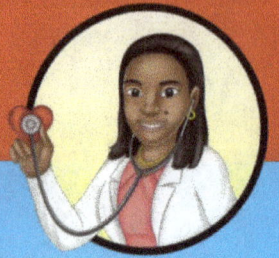

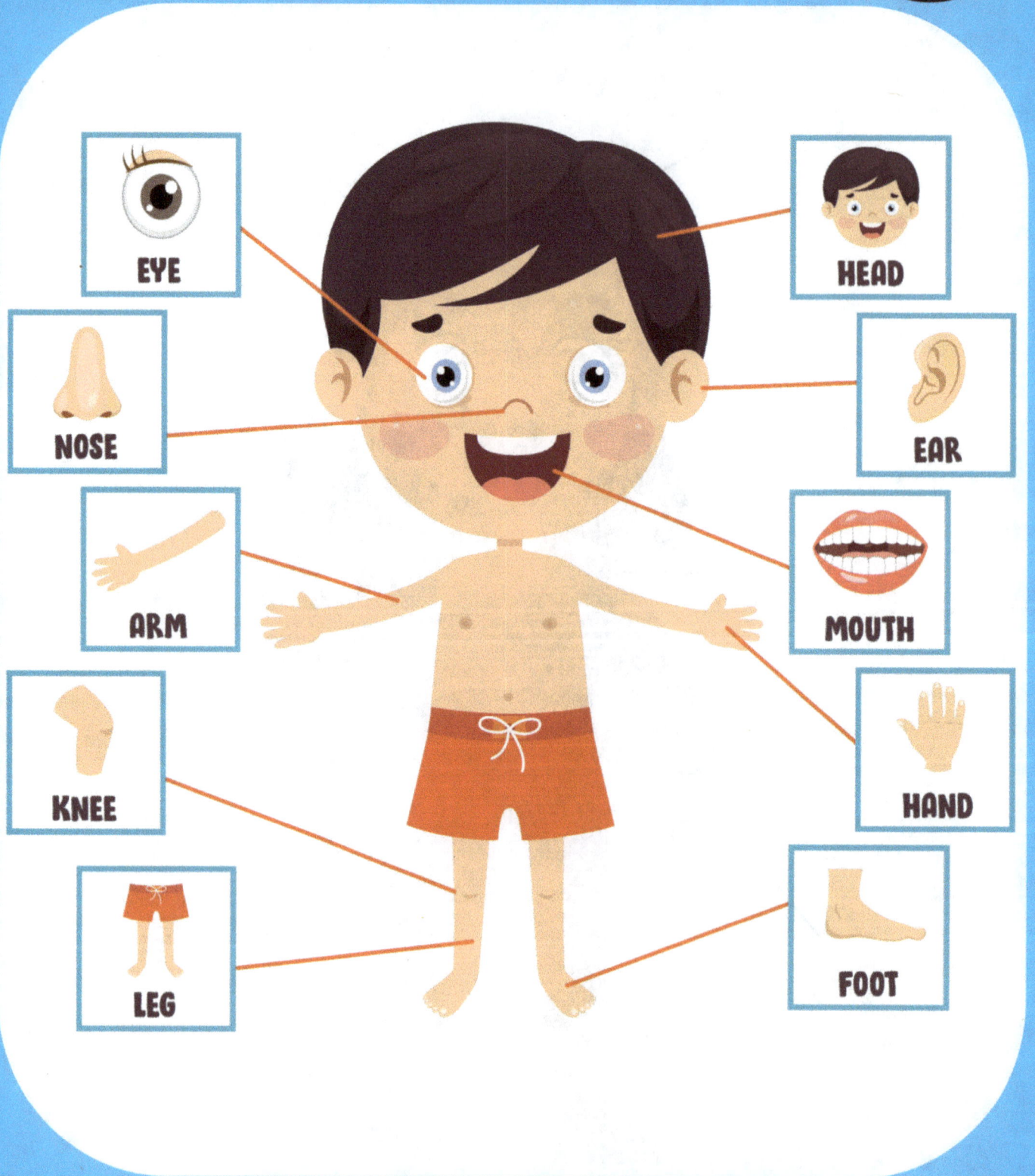

EYE

HEAD

NOSE

EAR

ARM

MOUTH

KNEE

HAND

LEG

FOOT

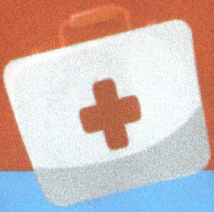

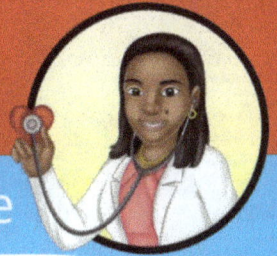

Connect the dots and color the picture

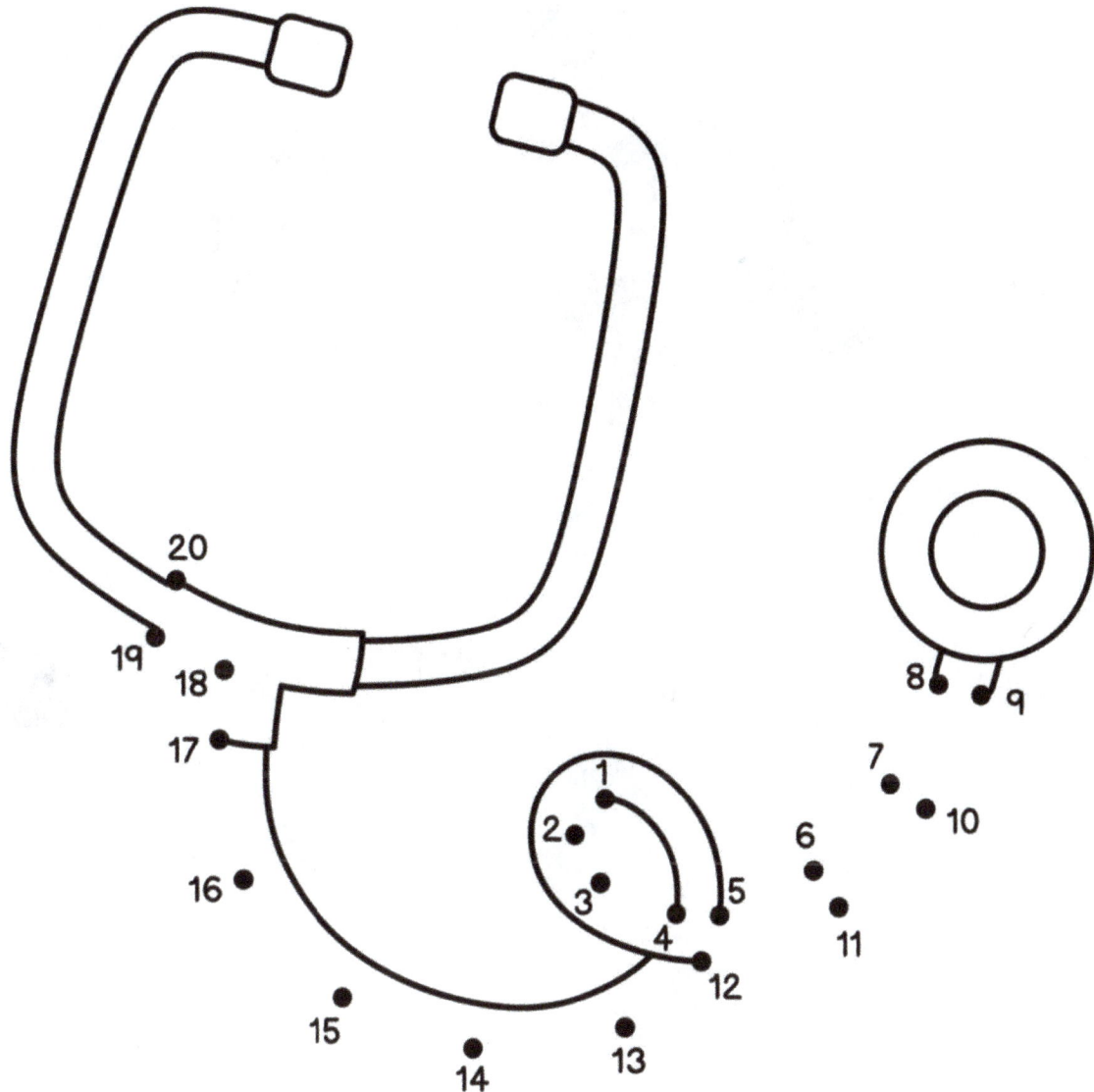

20

19

18

17

16

15

14

13

12

11

10

9

8

7

6

5

4

3

2

1

# HYGIENE

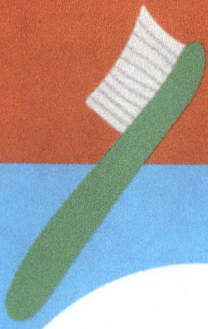

## How to brush your teeth

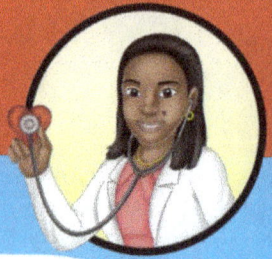

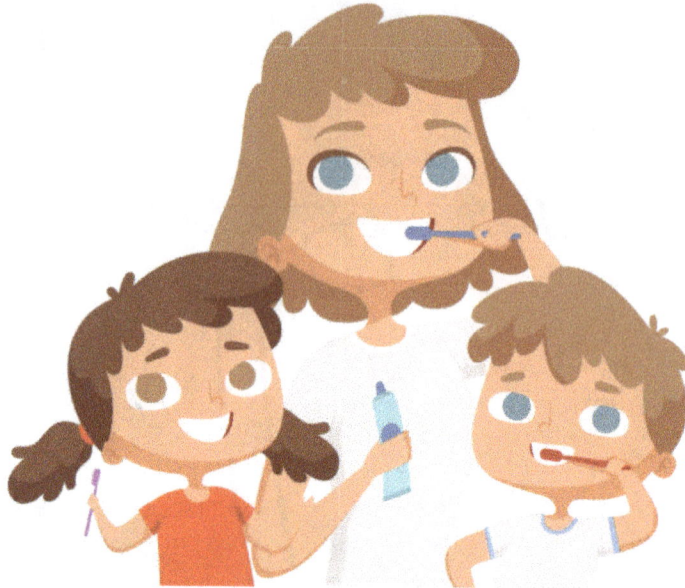

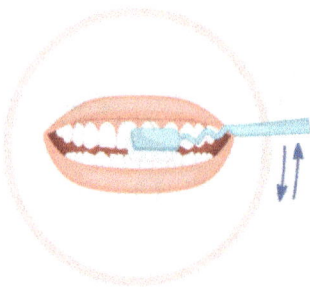

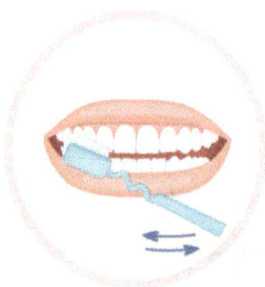

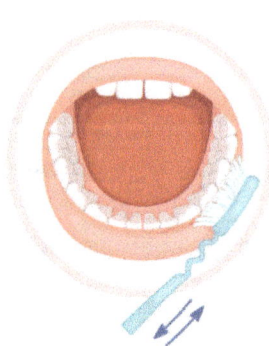

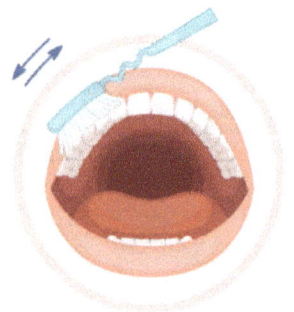

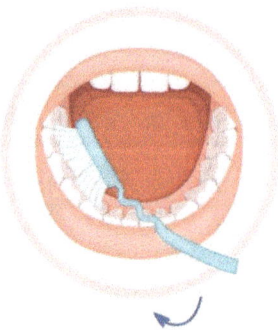

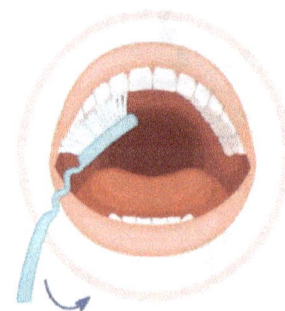

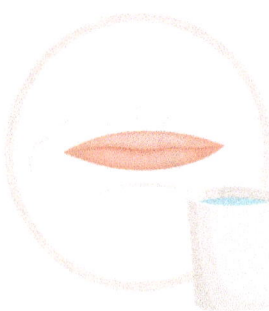

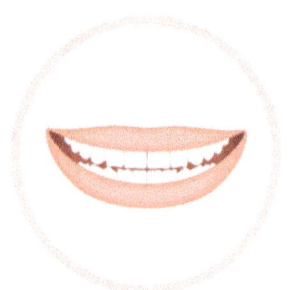

# MATCHING

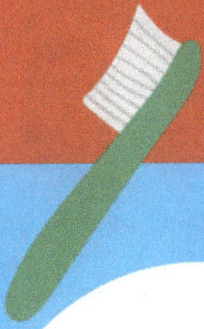

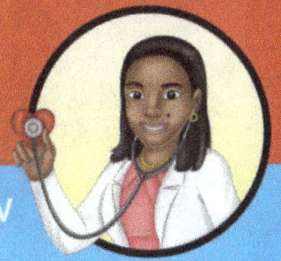

Match each picture with the correct shadow

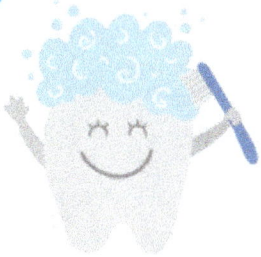

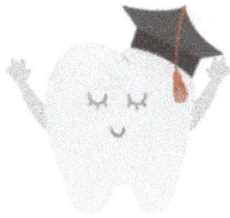

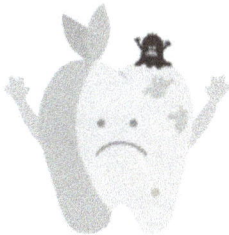

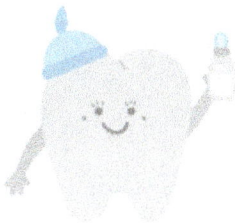

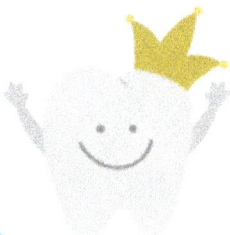

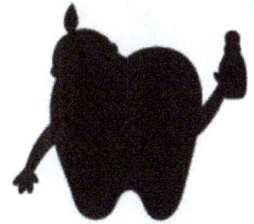

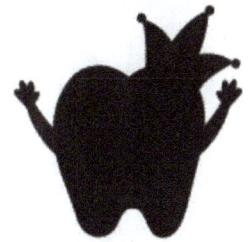

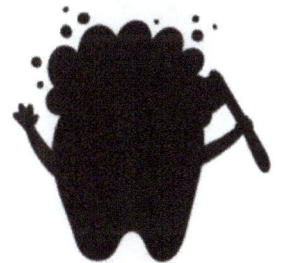

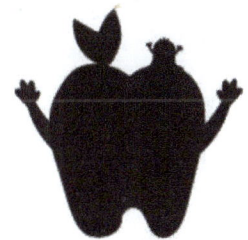

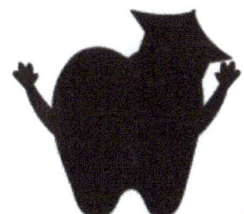

# 5 SENSES

Write the name of each sense

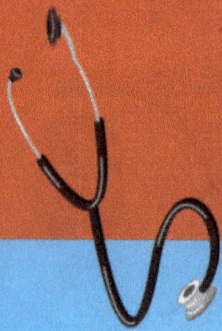
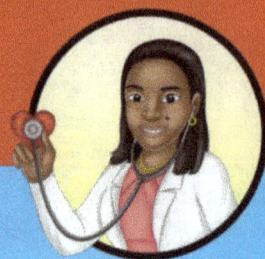
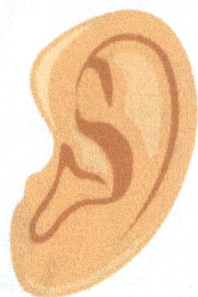
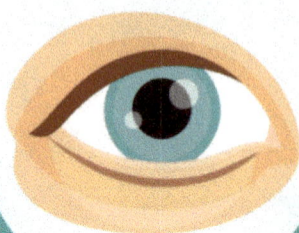
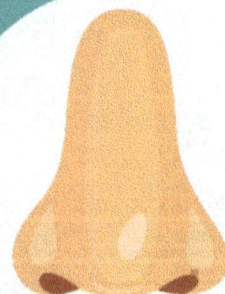
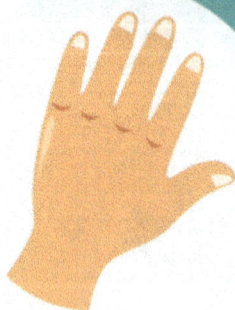
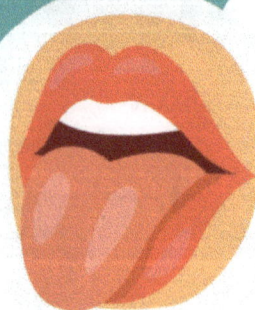

# MAZE

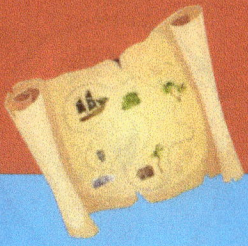

Help the boy find his ears

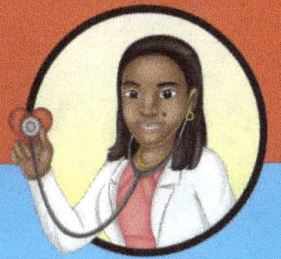

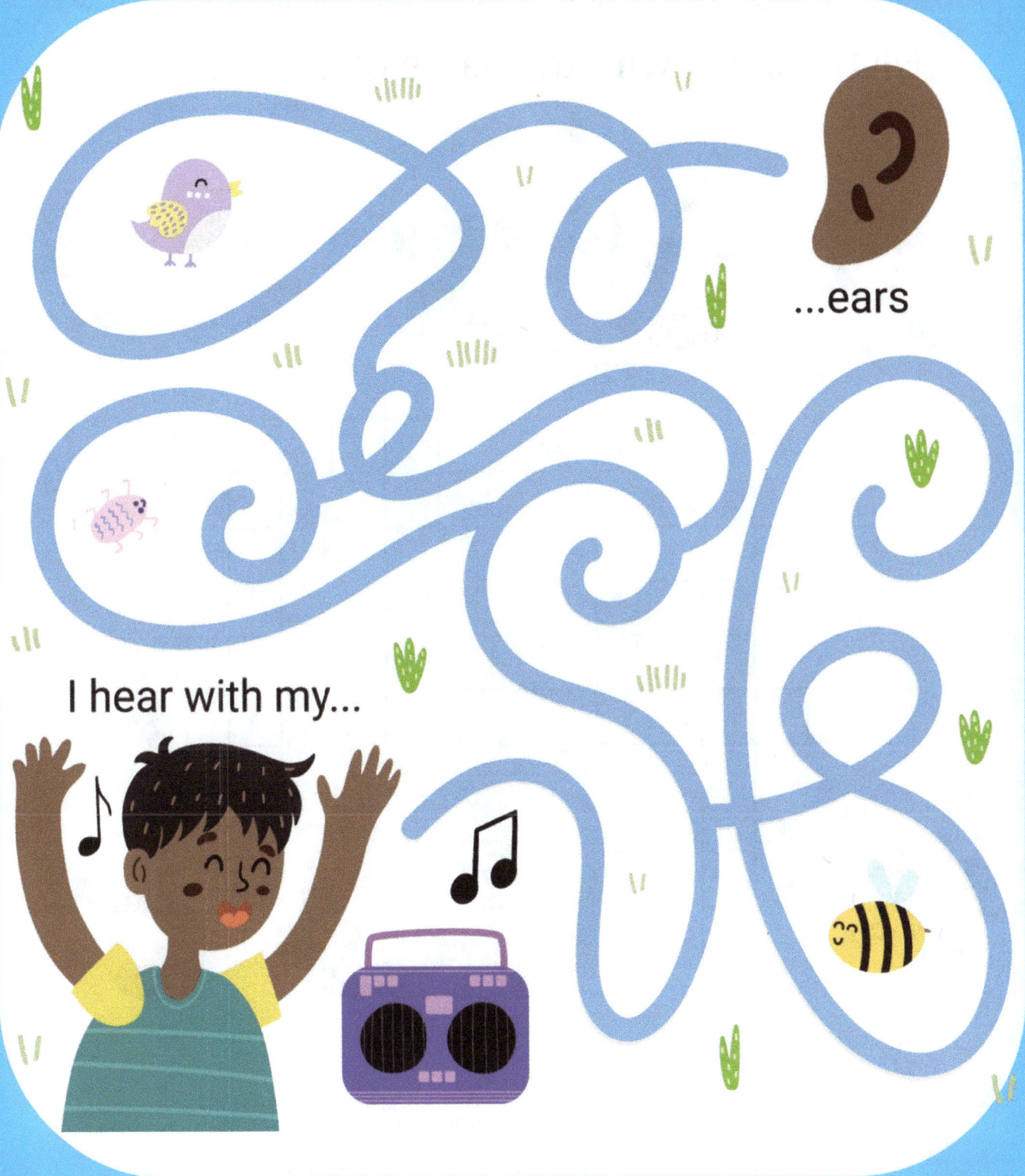

...ears

I hear with my...

# CROSSWORDS

## Fill the boxes with the name of each vegetable

1
2
3
4
5

6
7
8
9

1 Sweet Corn, 2 Pumpkin, 3 Broccoli, 4 Carrot, 7 Asparagus
5 Mushroom, 6 Kale, 8 Cauliflower, 9 Tomato

# HEALTHY FOOD

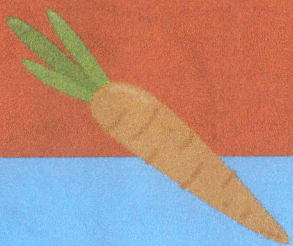

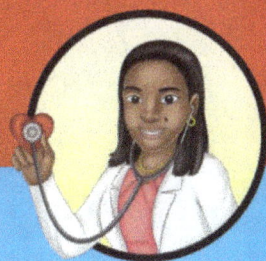

I eat healthy foods

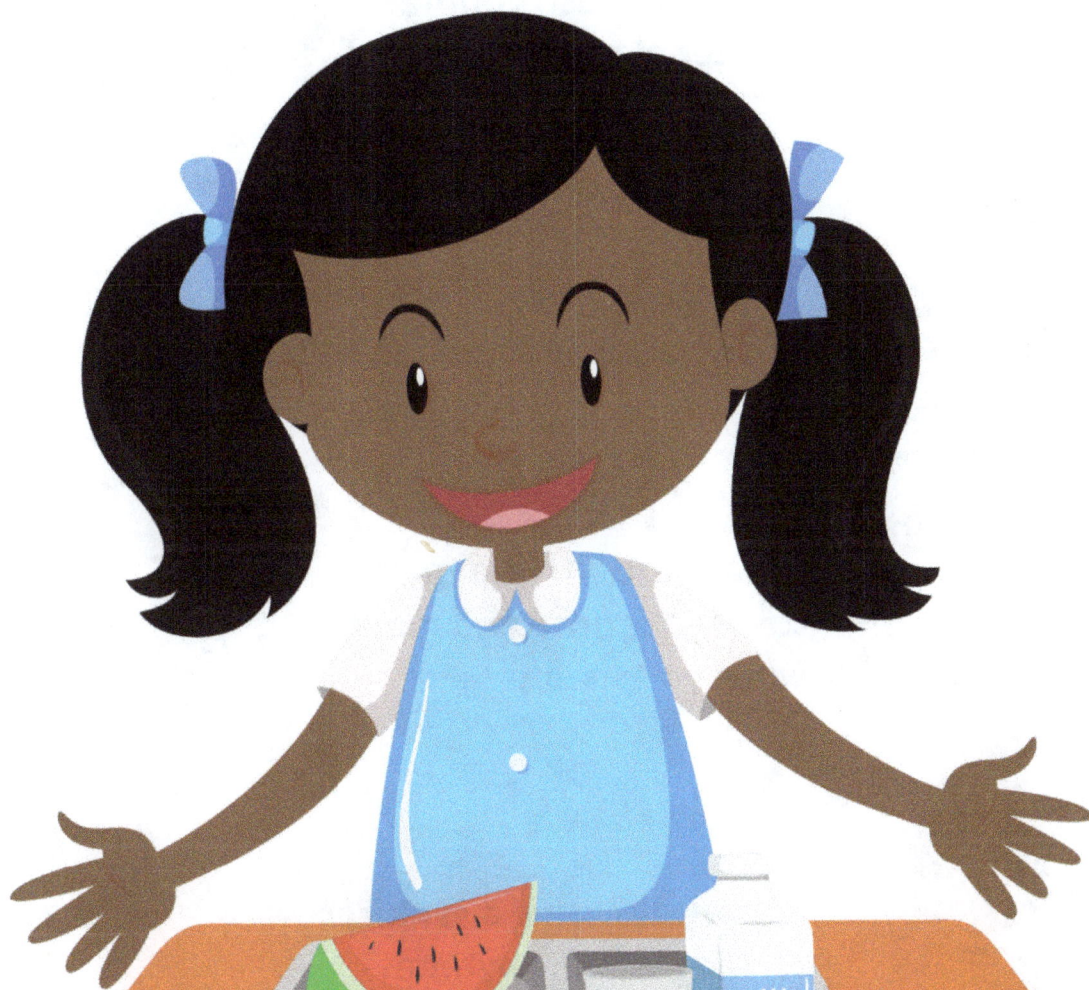

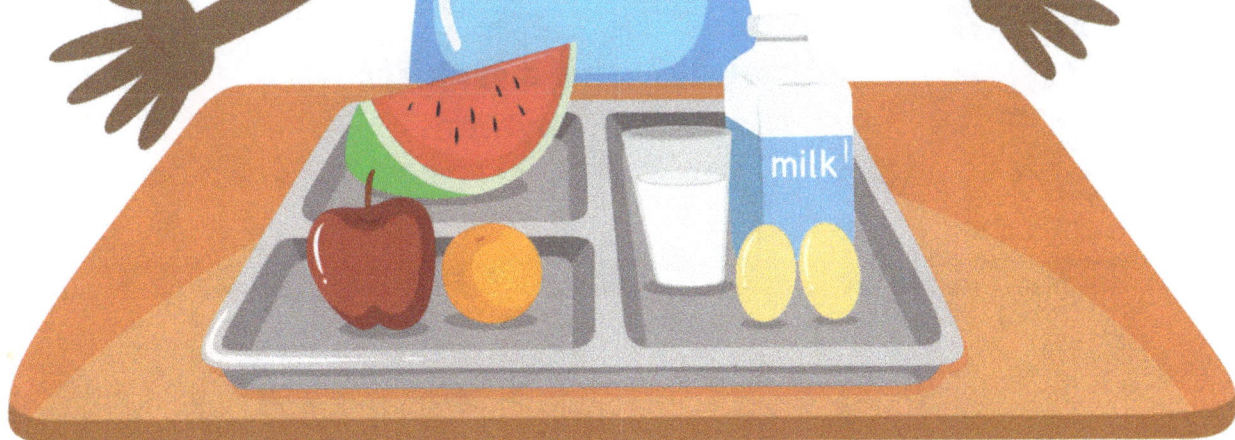

# HYGIENE

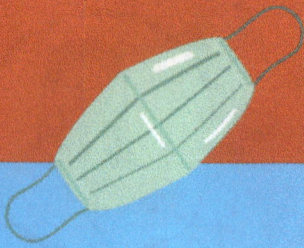

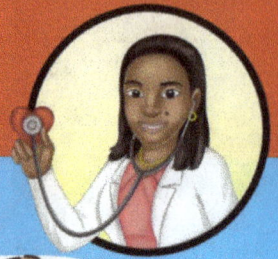

Always wash your feet after playing outside

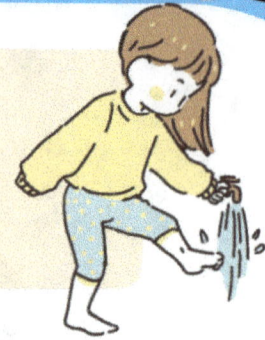

Always wash your hands before and after an activity

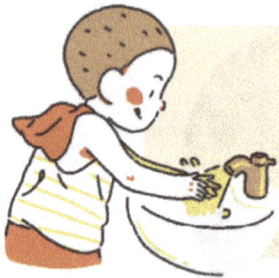

Always use a tissue to cover your nose and mouth when you sneeze

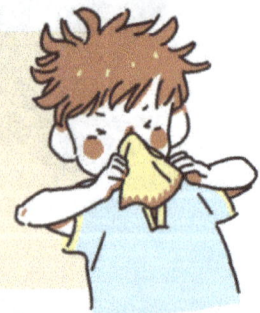

Always bring a sanitizer anywhere, anytime

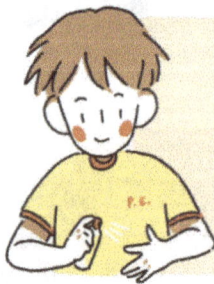

Always use your hand sanitizer

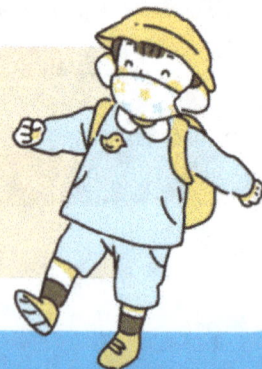

# HUMAN BODY

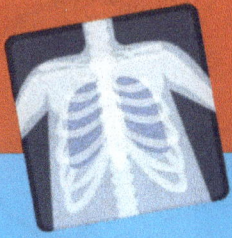
eye

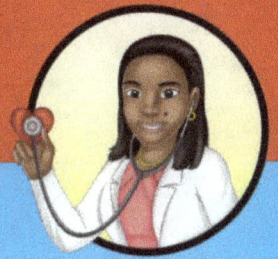

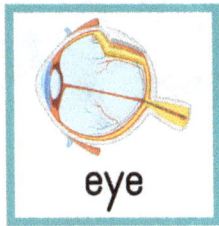
lungs

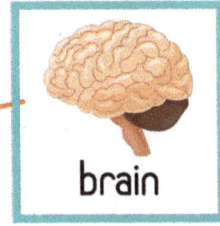
brain

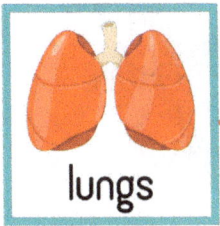
liver

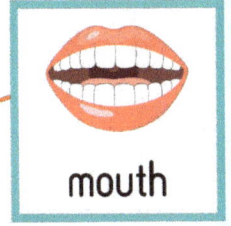
mouth

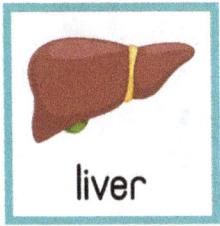
kidney

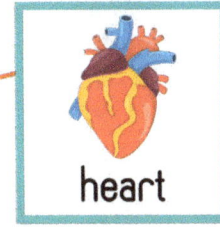
heart

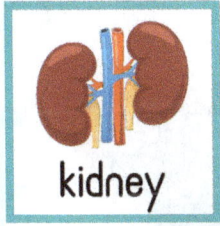
spleen

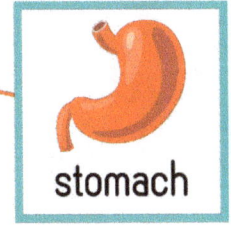
stomach

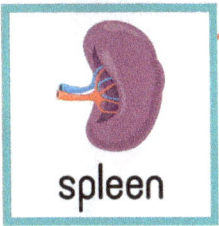

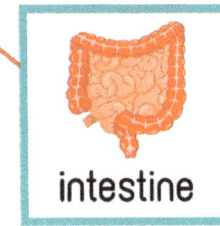
intestine

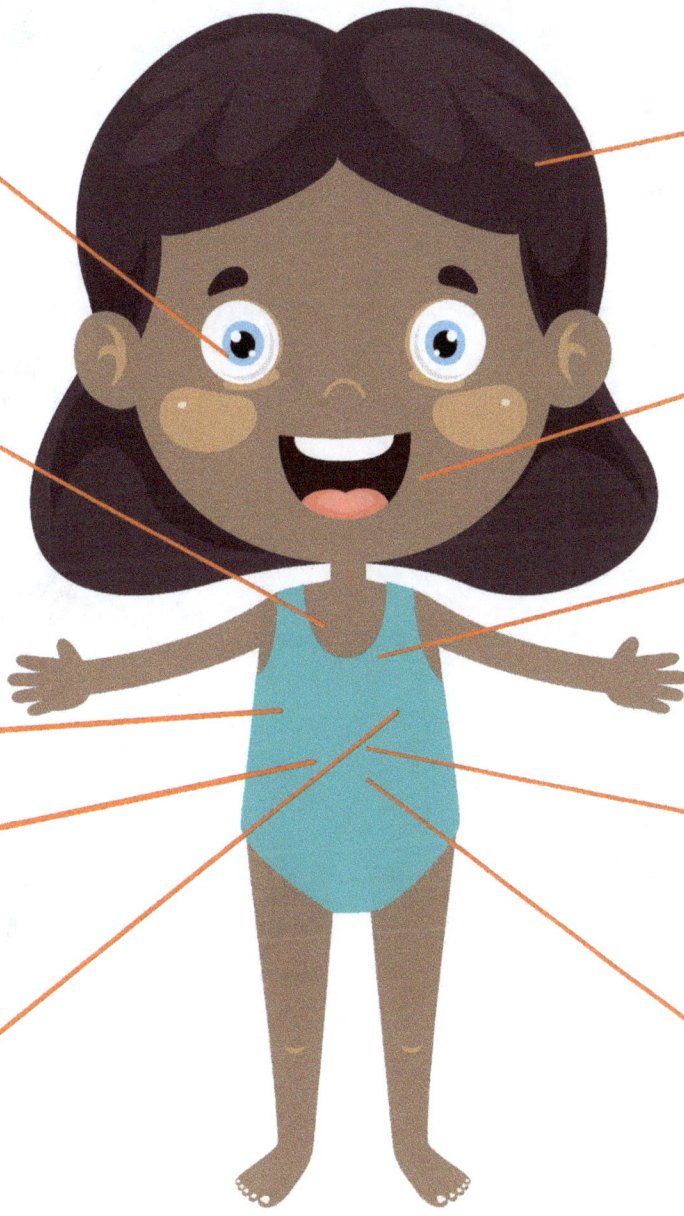

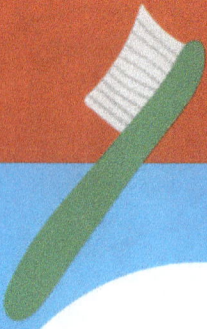

# MATCHING

Match with the correct number

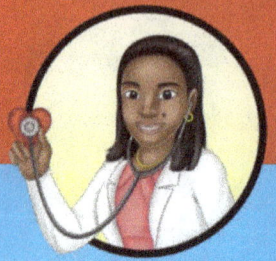

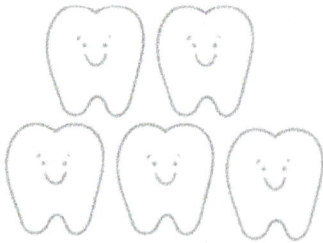
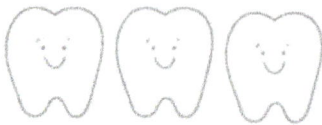

3

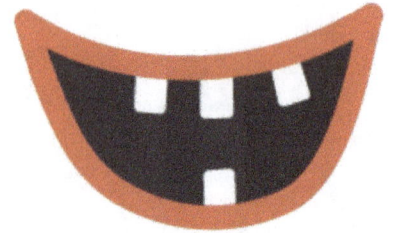

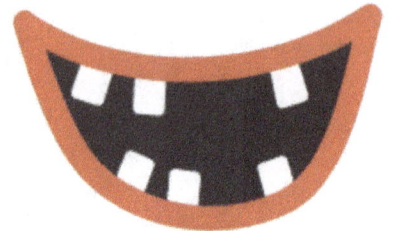

7

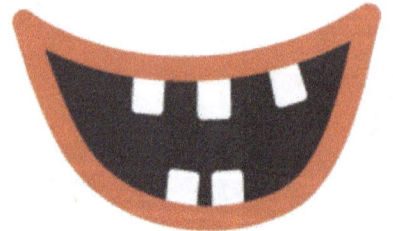

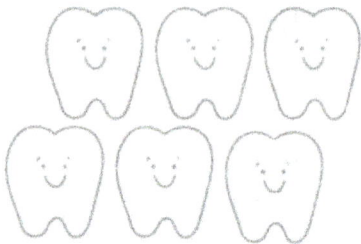

4

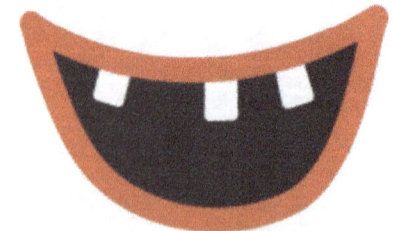

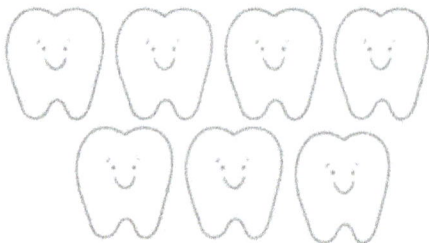

5

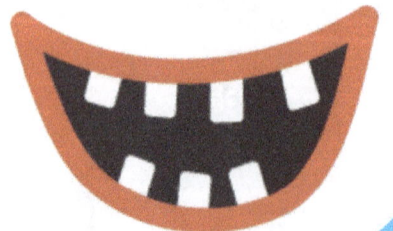

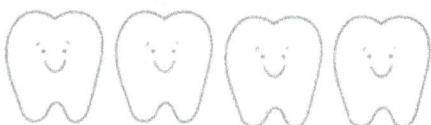

6

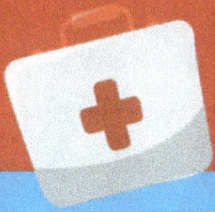
# CONNECTING DOTS
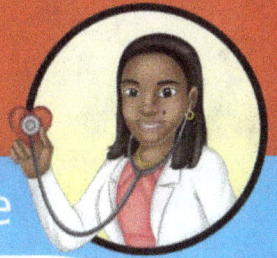

Connect the dots and color the picture

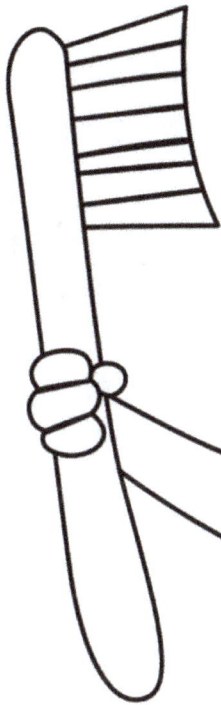

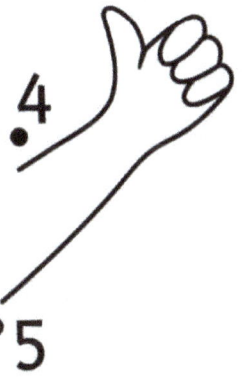

18

1

2

17

3

16

4

15

5

14

6

10

13

11

7

9

12

8

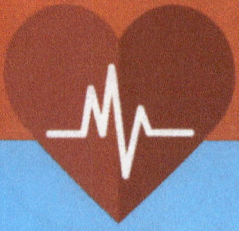

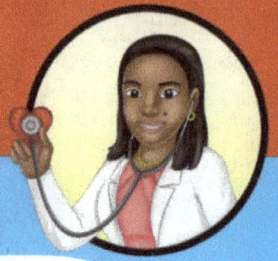

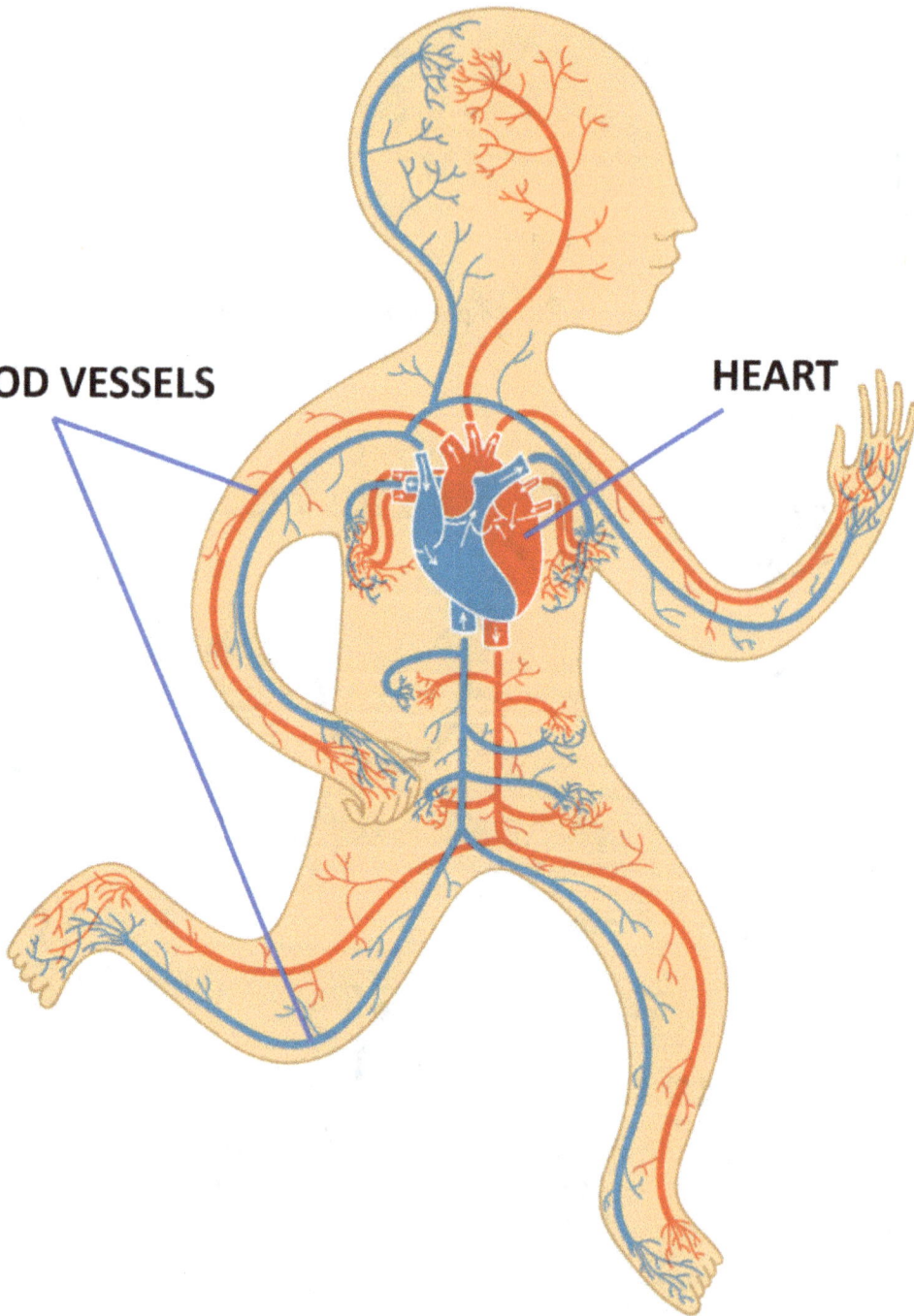

BLOOD VESSELS

HEART

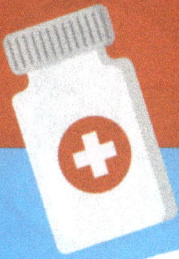
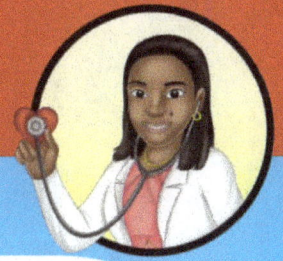

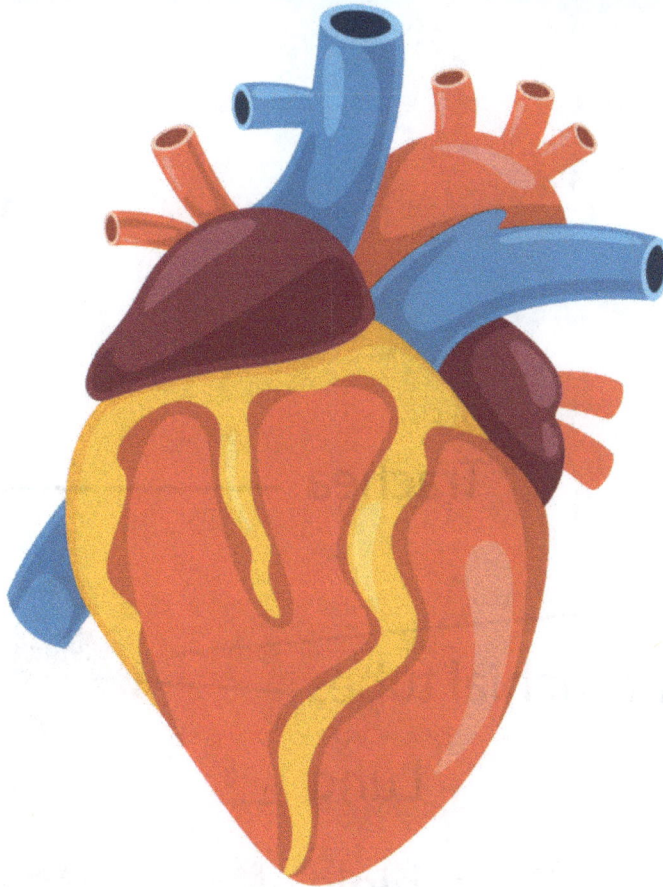

# HEART

The heart is the organ, or body part, that pumps blood through the body. It is the main organ of the cardiovascular system. The cardiovascular system carries substances to and from all parts of the body in the blood.

# RESPIRATORY SYSTEM

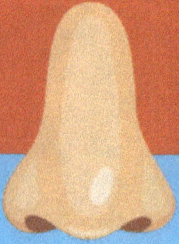

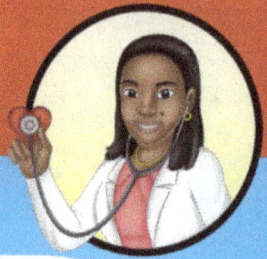

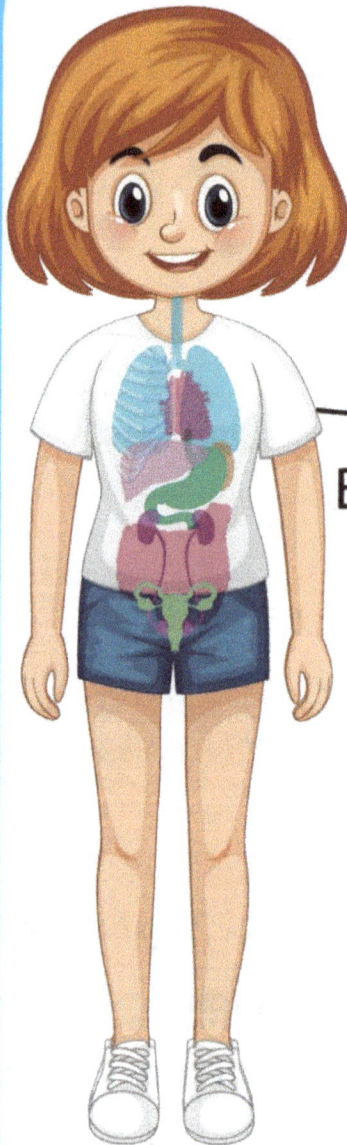

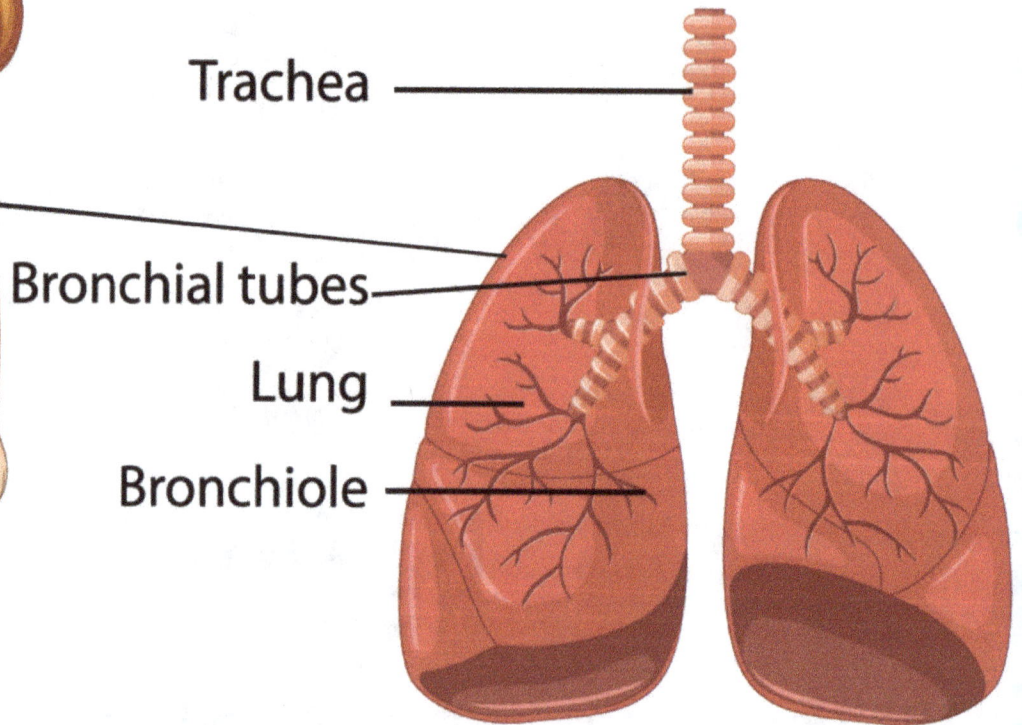

Trachea

Bronchial tubes

Lung

Bronchiole

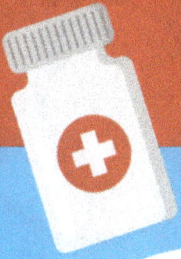
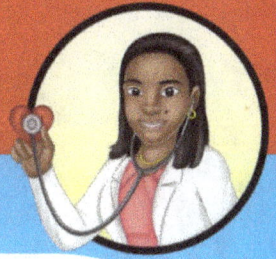

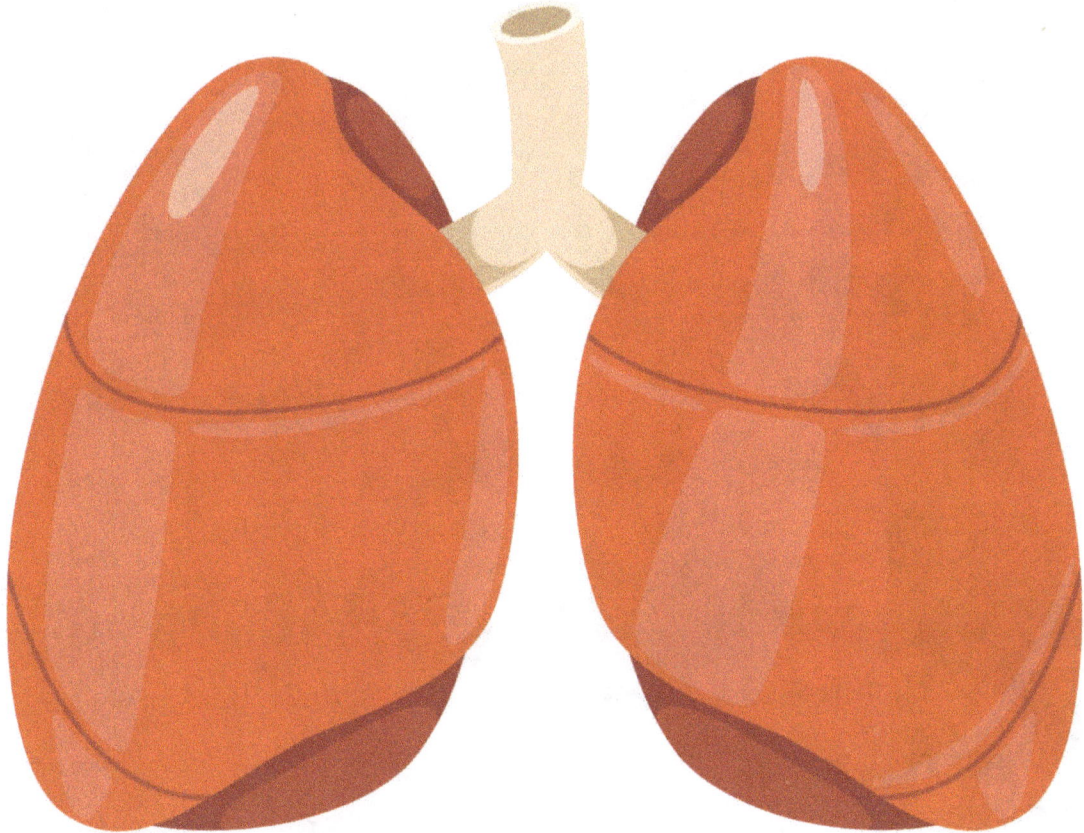

# LUNGS

The lungs are a pair of spongy air filled organs on either side of the chest. They are used for breathing and form part of the respiratory system.

# BREATHING

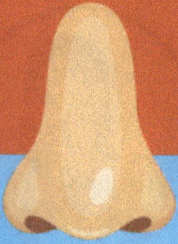

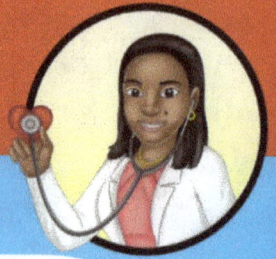

## This is how the lungs work

### Breathing in

Trachea

Lungs

Diaphragm

**Inhalation**

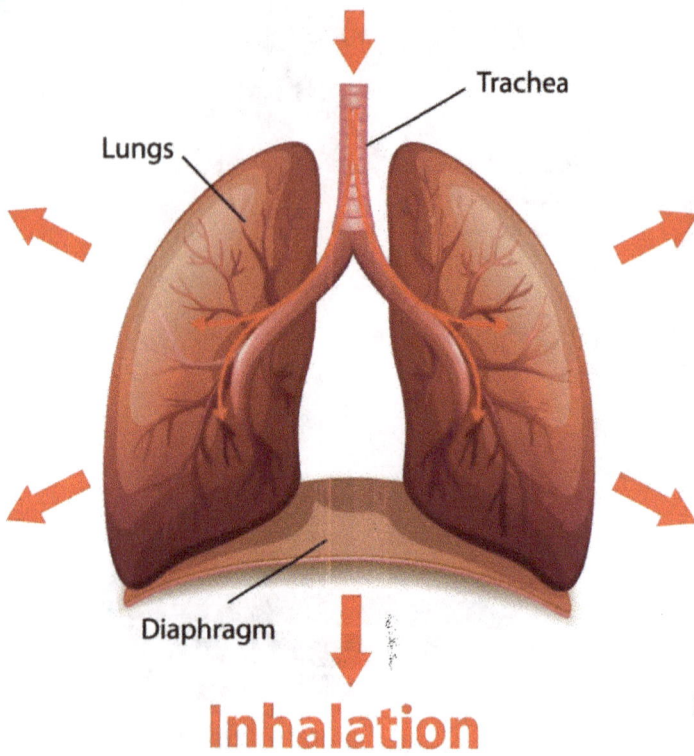

### Breathing out

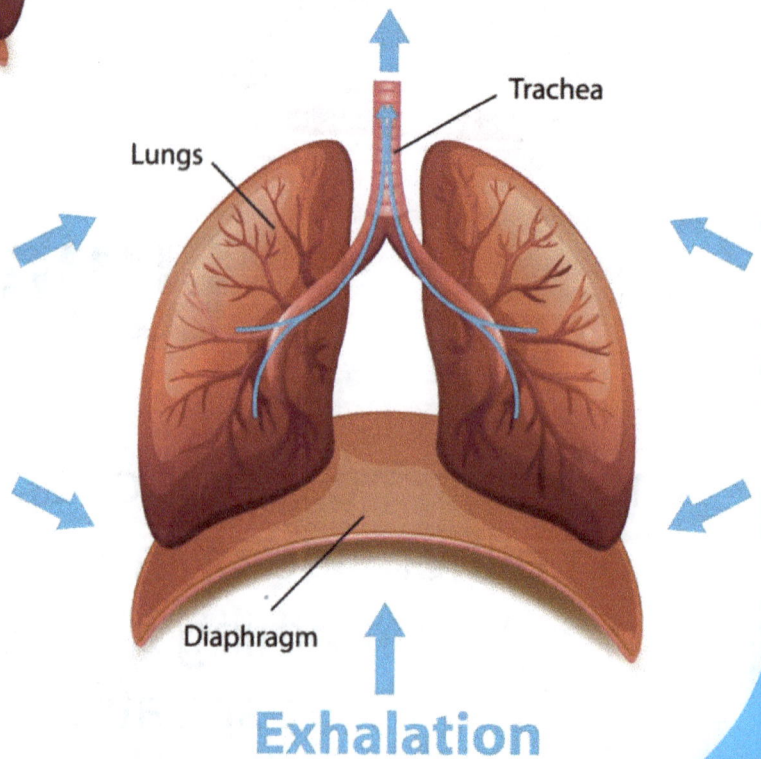

Lungs

Trachea

Diaphragm

**Exhalation**

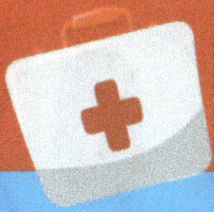

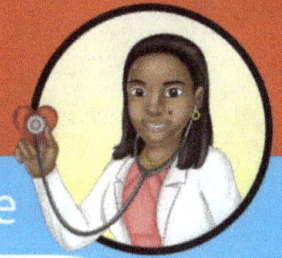

Connect the dots and color the picture

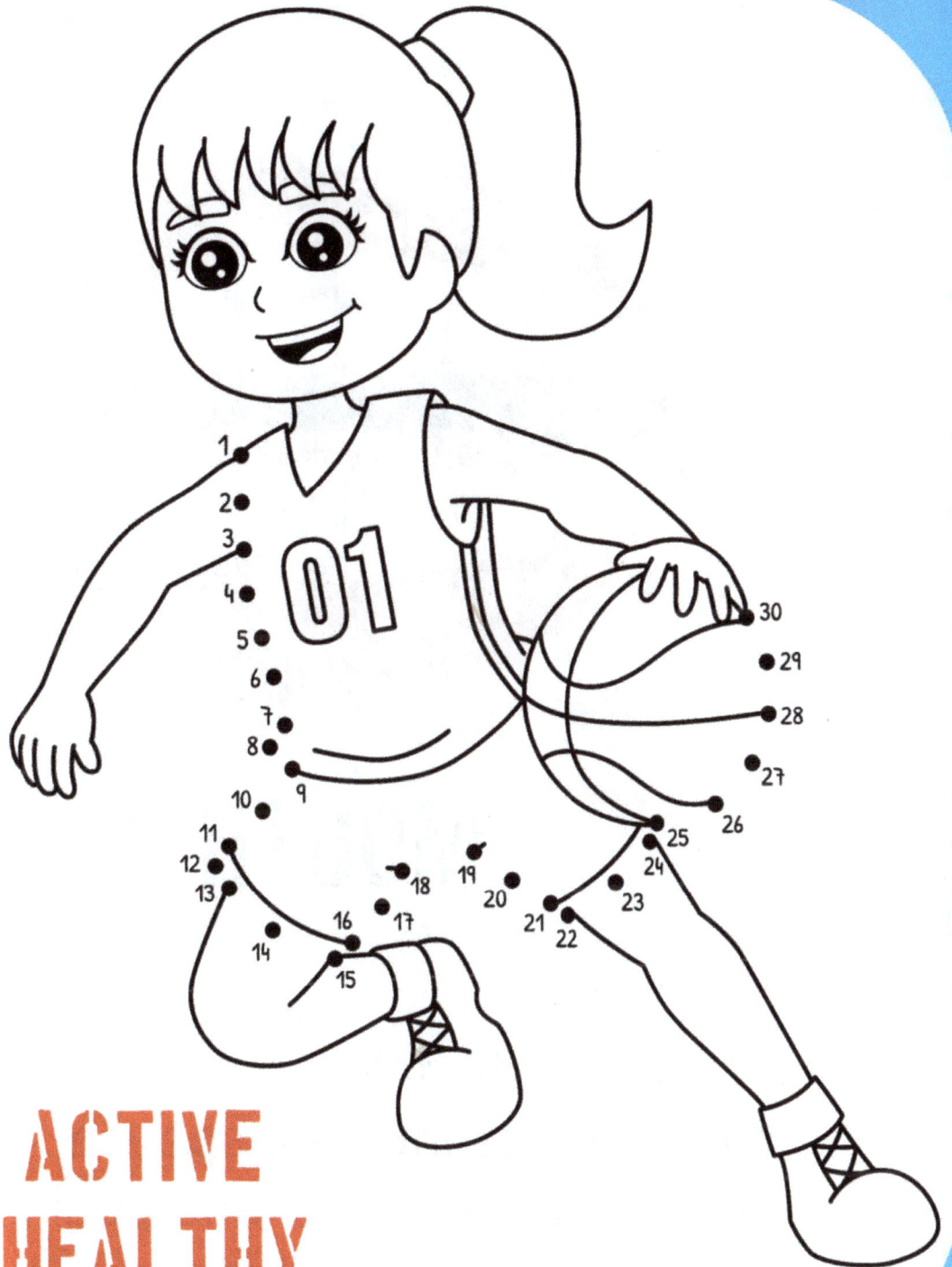

**STAY ACTIVE
STAY HEALTHY**

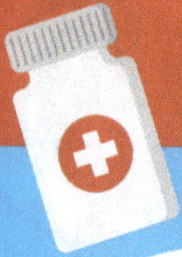
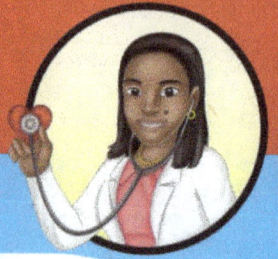

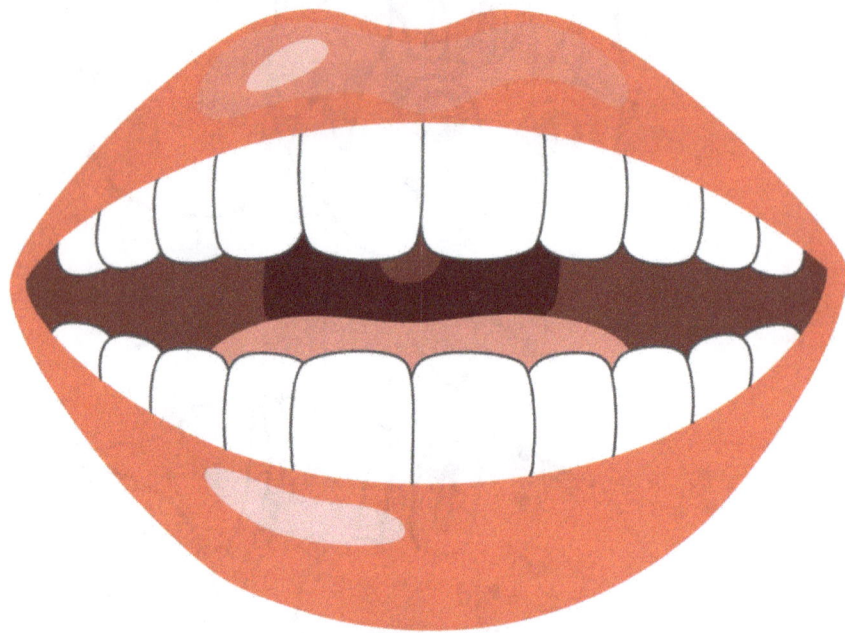

# MOUTH

Every time we smile, talk or eat we use our mouth. The mouth is essential for speech. Our mouth lets us eat and drink and begins the process of digestion.

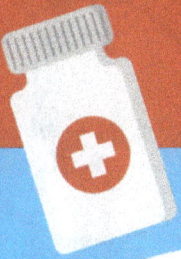
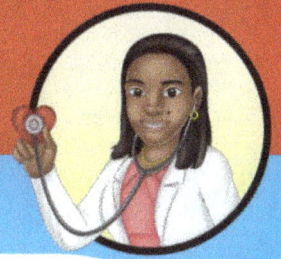

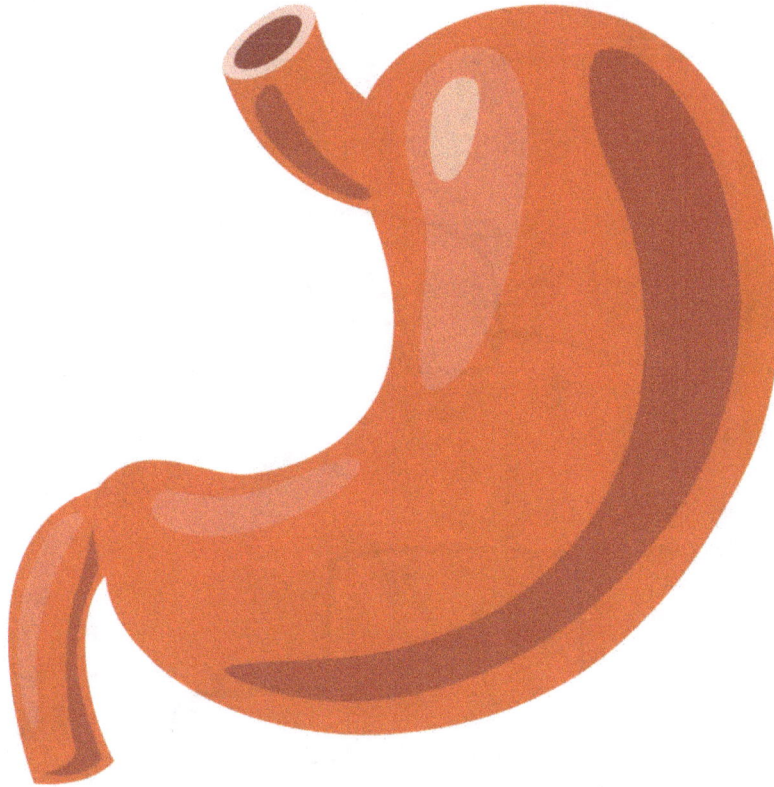

# STOMACH

The stomach is a hollow organ and forms a part of the digestive system. Food lands in the stomach after passing down the throat through a tube called the esophagus. The stomach is like a balloon and stores our food and passes it along in small amounts to the small intestines.

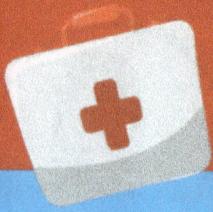

# CONNECTING DOTS

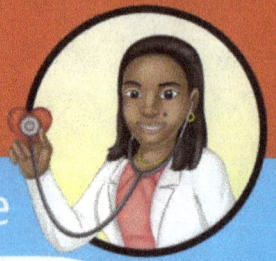

Connect the dots and color the picture

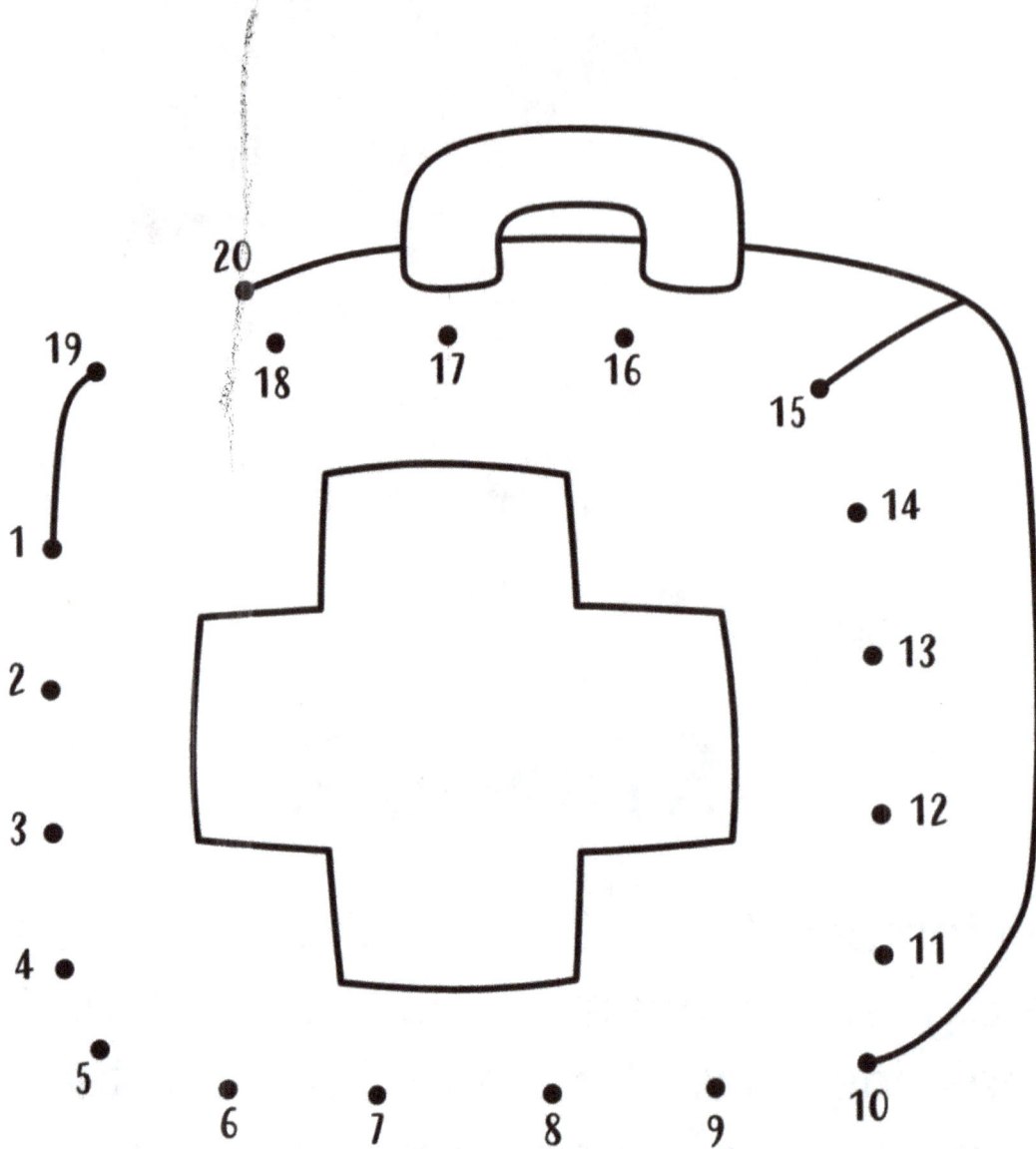

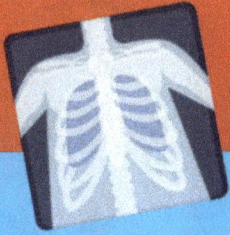

# HUMAN BODY

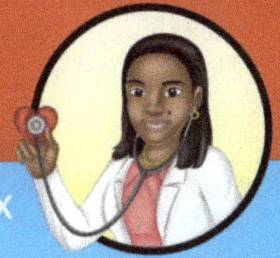

write name of organ/body part in each box

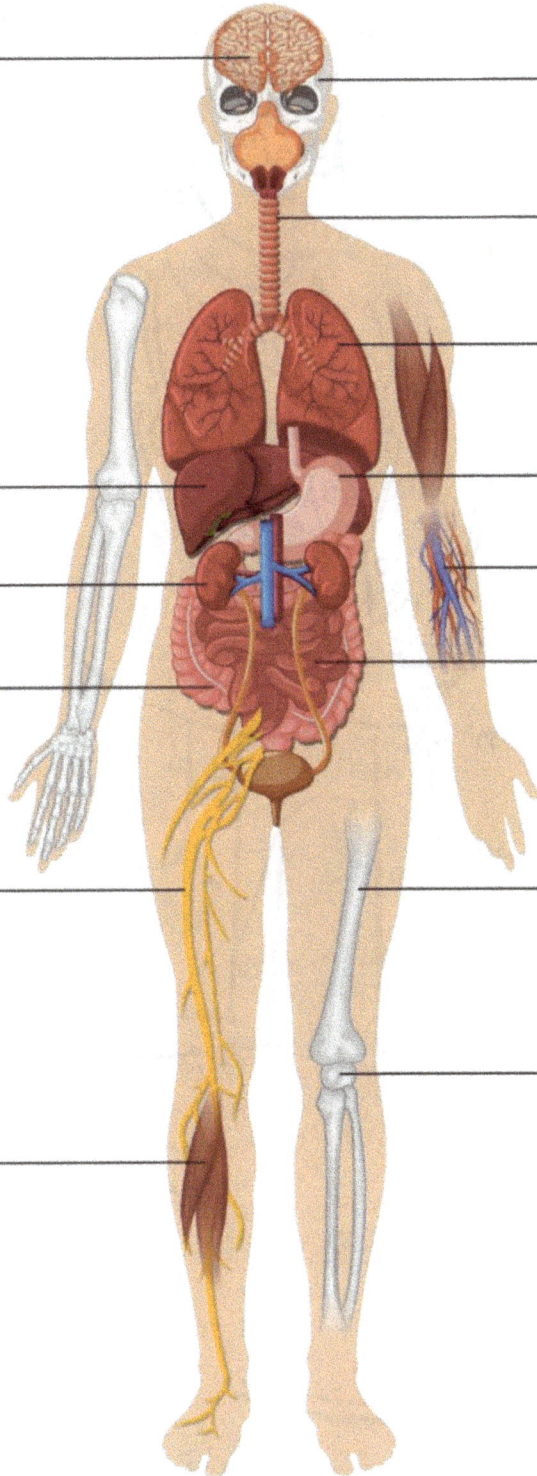

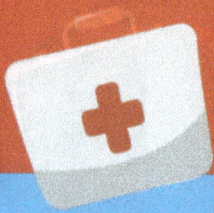

# CONNECTING DOTS

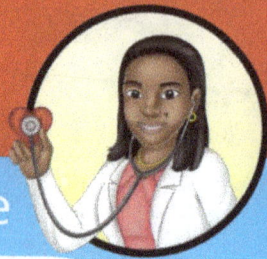

Connect the dots and color the picture

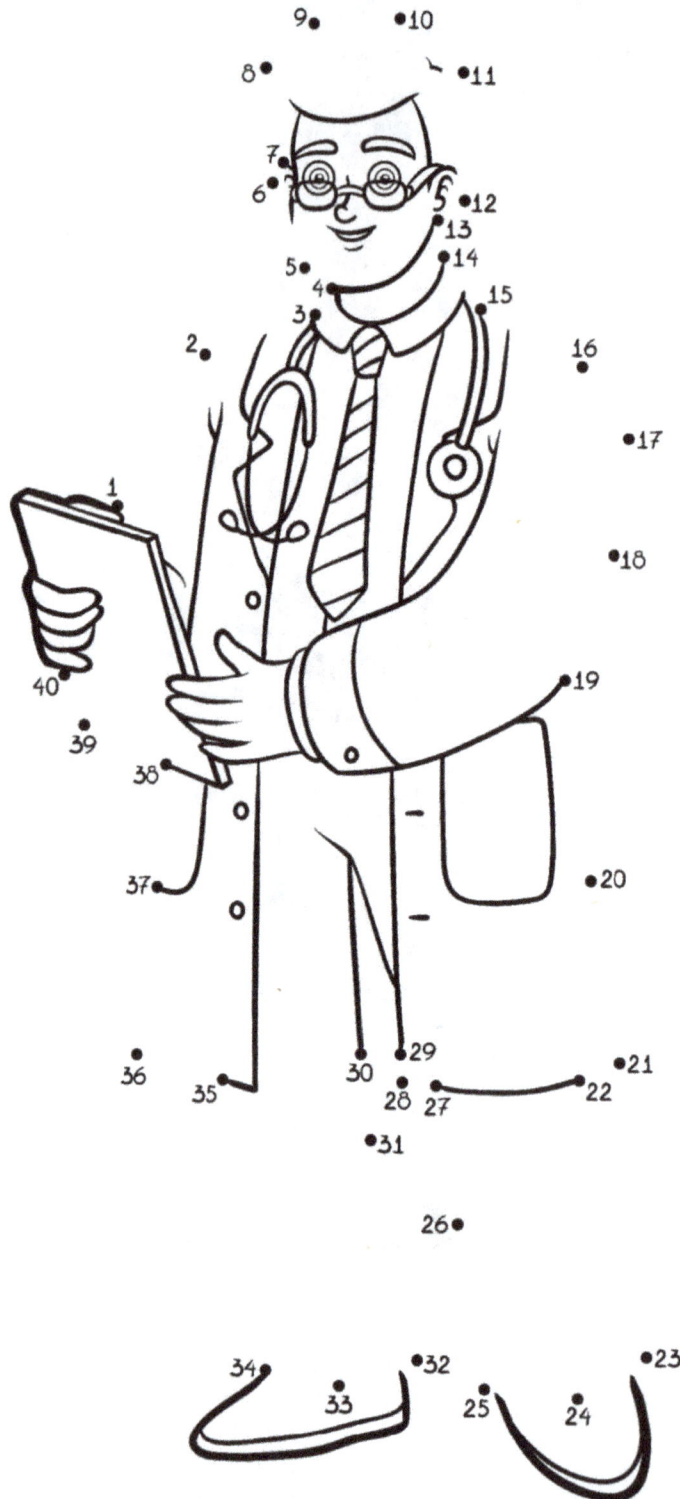

# DIGESTIVE SYSTEM

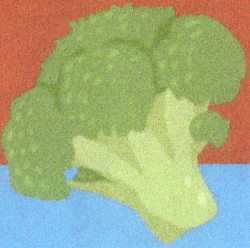

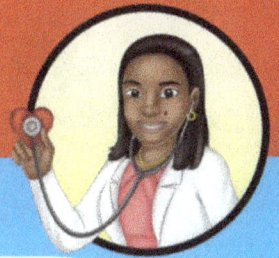

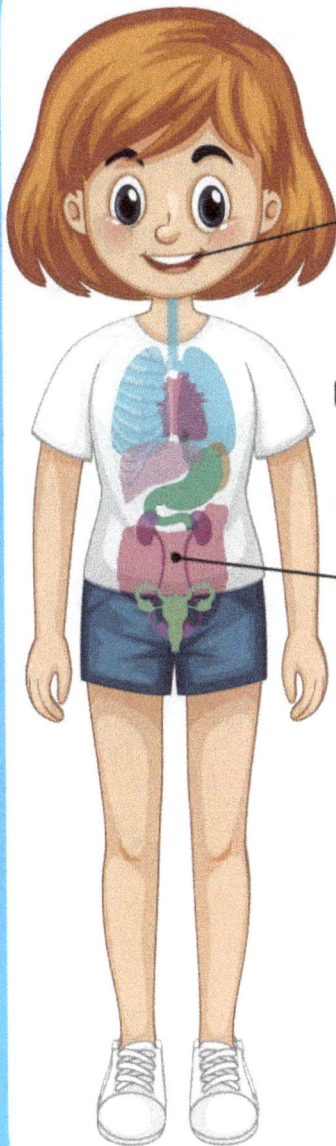

ORAL CAVITY

ESOPHAGUS

LIVER

GALLBLADDER

STOMACH

PANCREAS

LARGE
INTESTINE

SMALL
INTESTINE

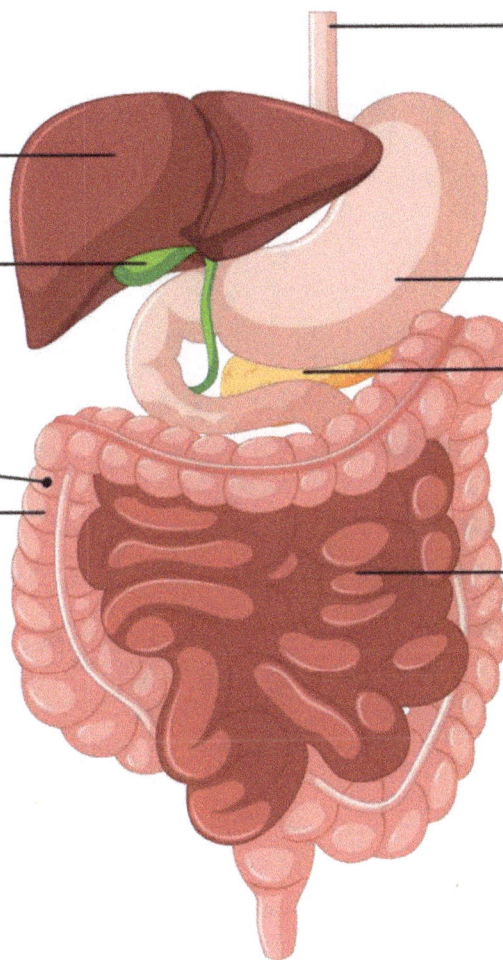

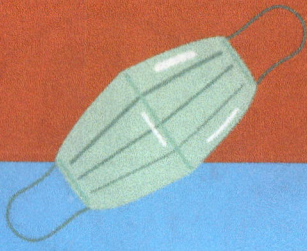

# HYGIENE

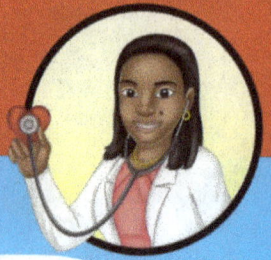

## How to wash your hands

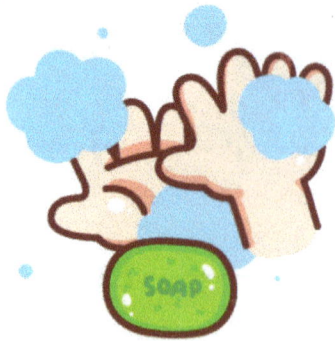

**USE SOAP**

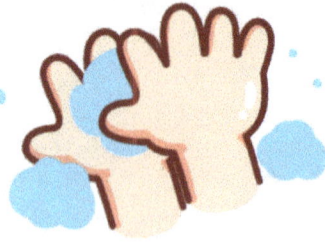

**WASH**

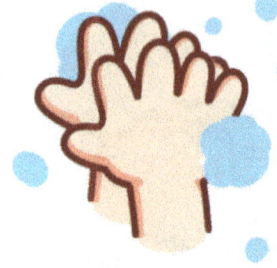

**BETWEEN FINGERS**

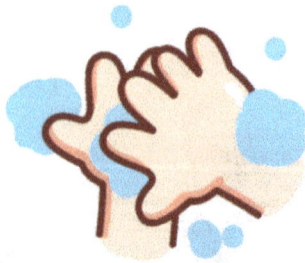

**BACK OF HANDS**

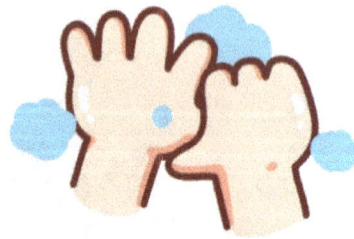

**THUMBS**

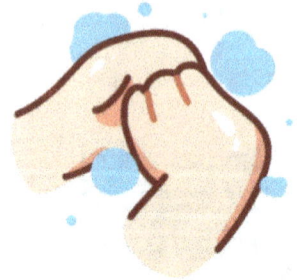

**BACK OF FINGERS**

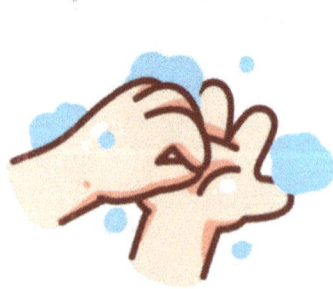

**FINGERNAILS**

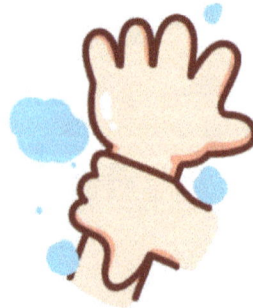

**WRISTS**

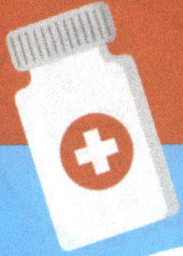
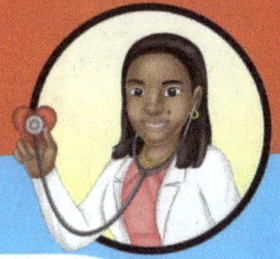

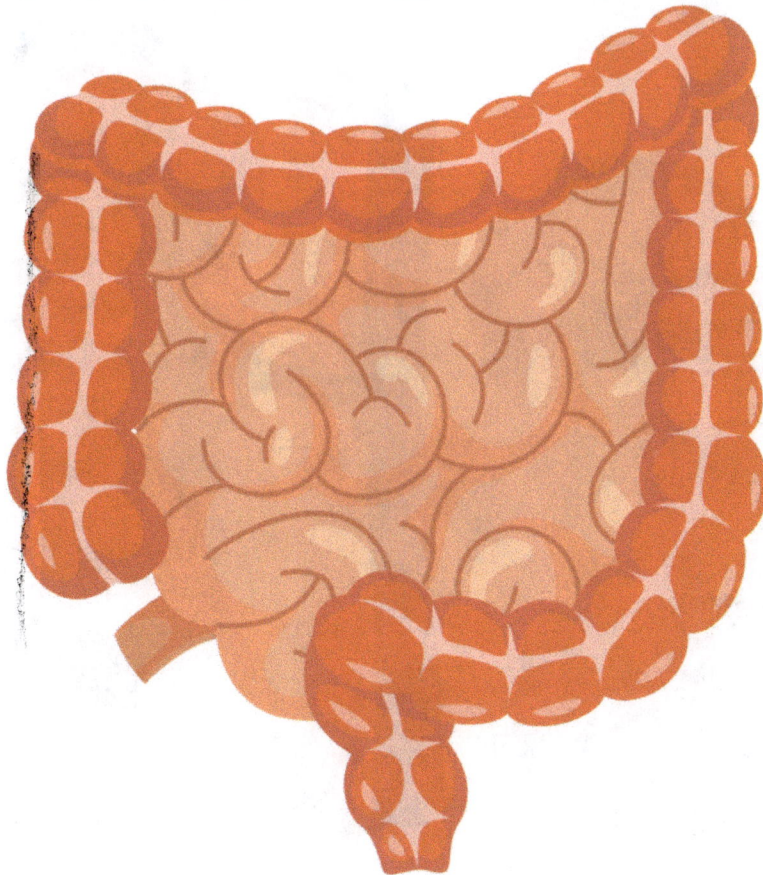

# INTESTINE

The intestines are organs, or body parts, that are shaped like long tubes. They help break down food so that the body can use it for energy. This is part of the process called digestion. The intestines also remove wastes from the body.

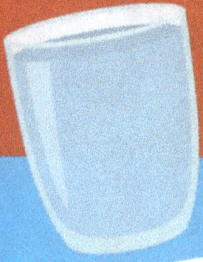
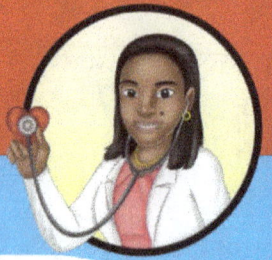

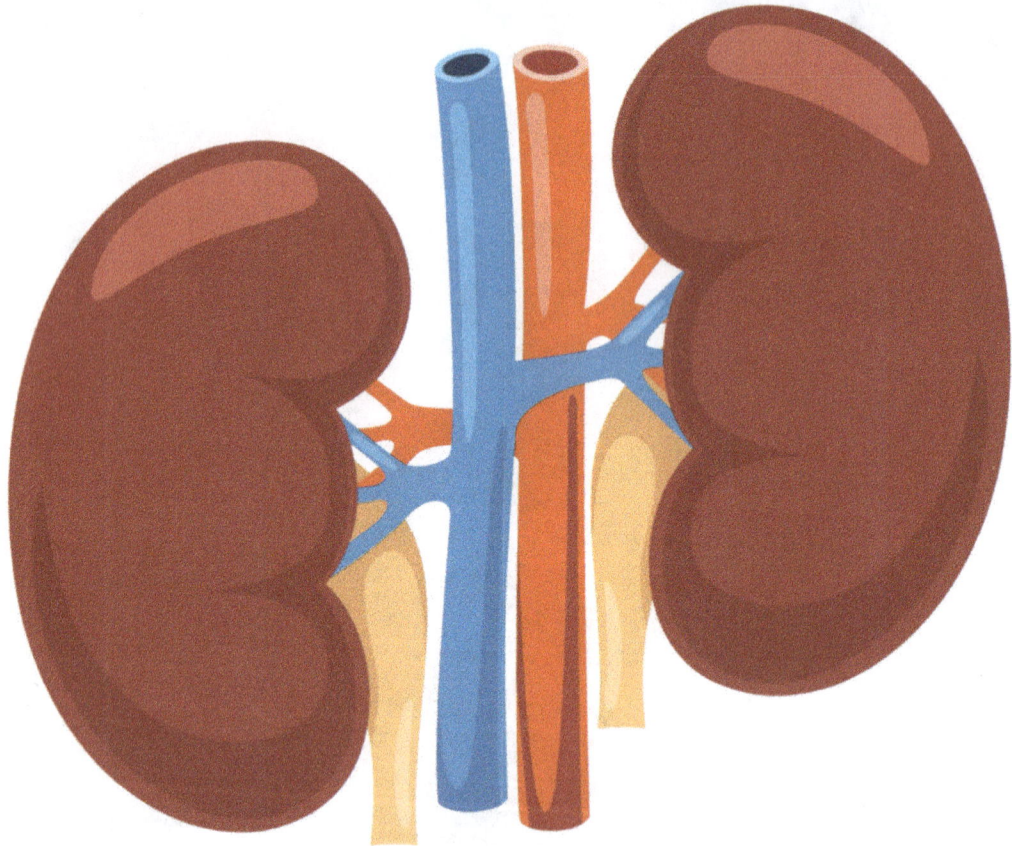

# KIDNEY

The kidneys are a pair of organs that are found on either side of the spine, just below the rib cage in the back. Kidneys filter waste materials out of the blood and pass them out of the body as urine. We drink plenty of water to keep our kidneys happy. 😊

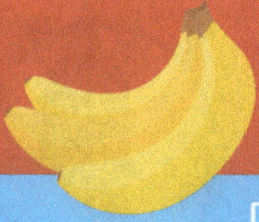

# HUMAN BODY

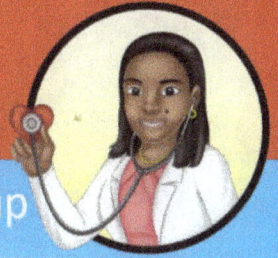

Draw and color at least 2 foods in each group

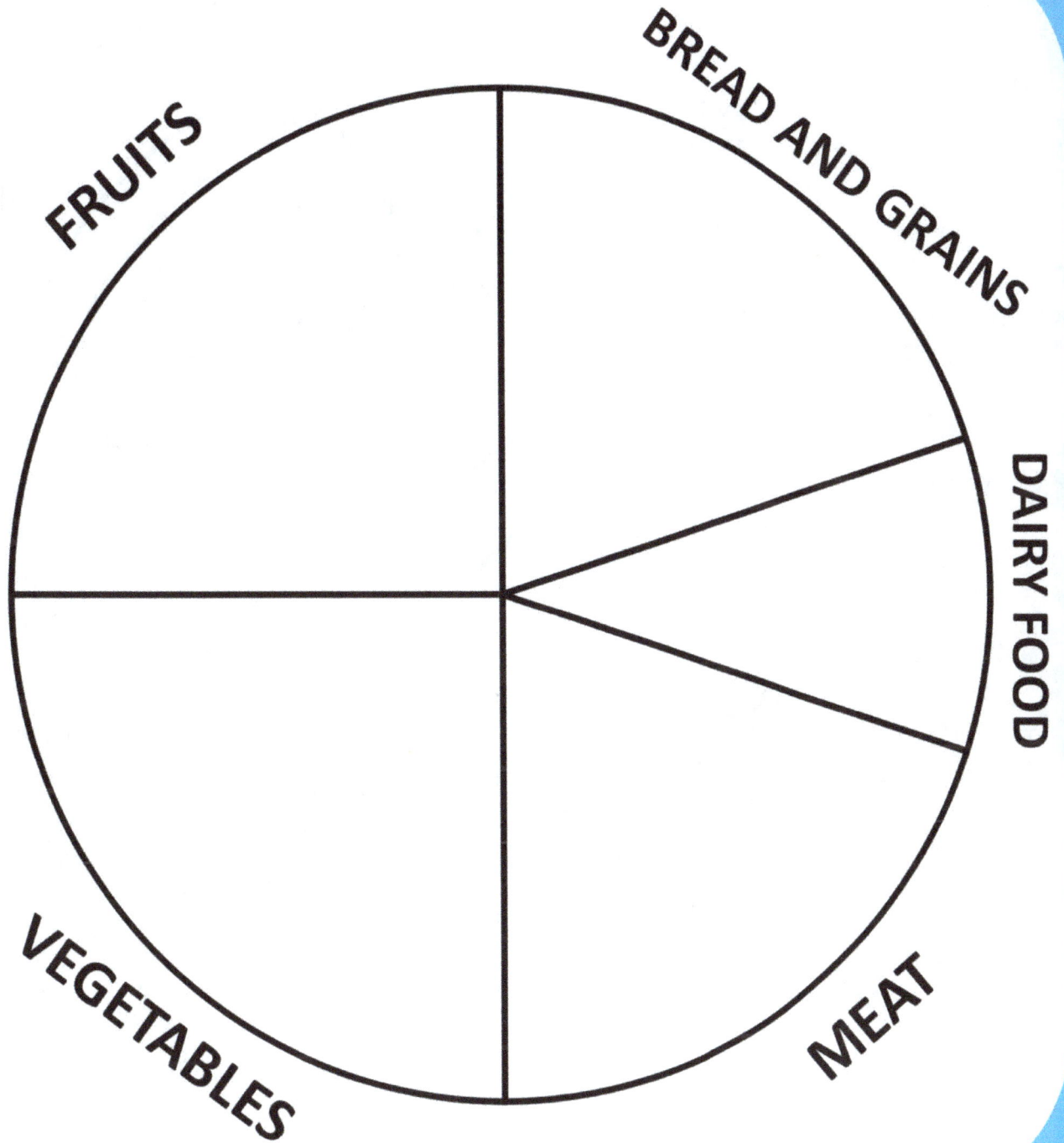

FRUITS

BREAD AND GRAINS

DAIRY FOOD

MEAT

VEGETABLES

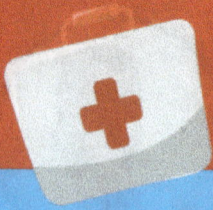

# CONNECTING DOTS

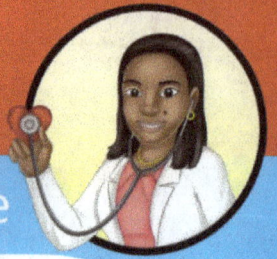

Connect the dots and color the picture

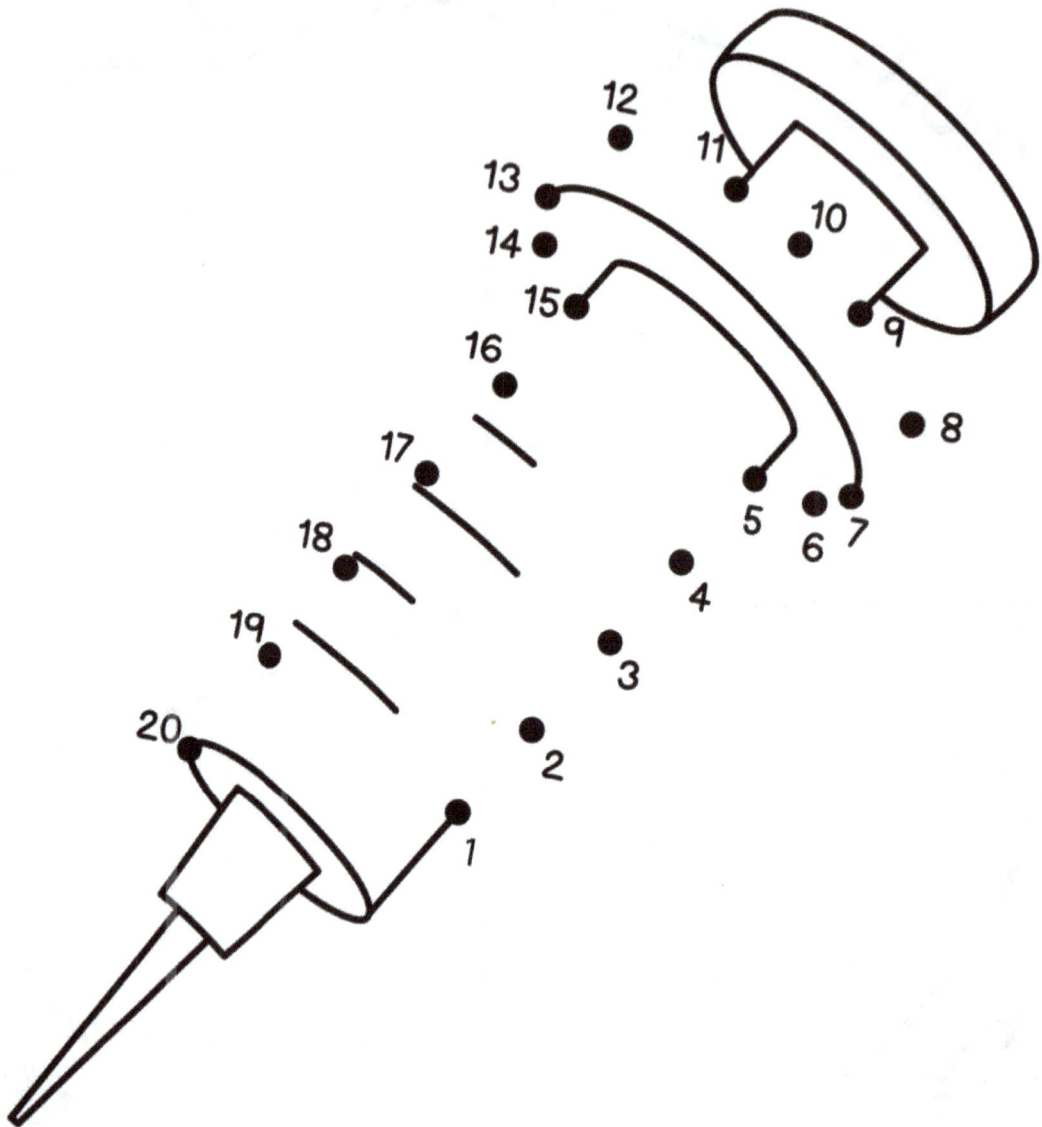

12
13
11
14
10
15
16
9
17
8
18
5 6 7
19
4
3
20
2
1

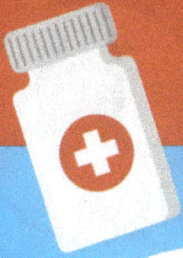
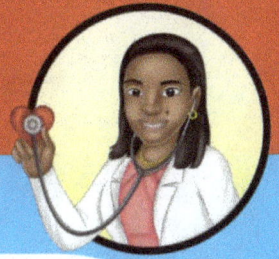

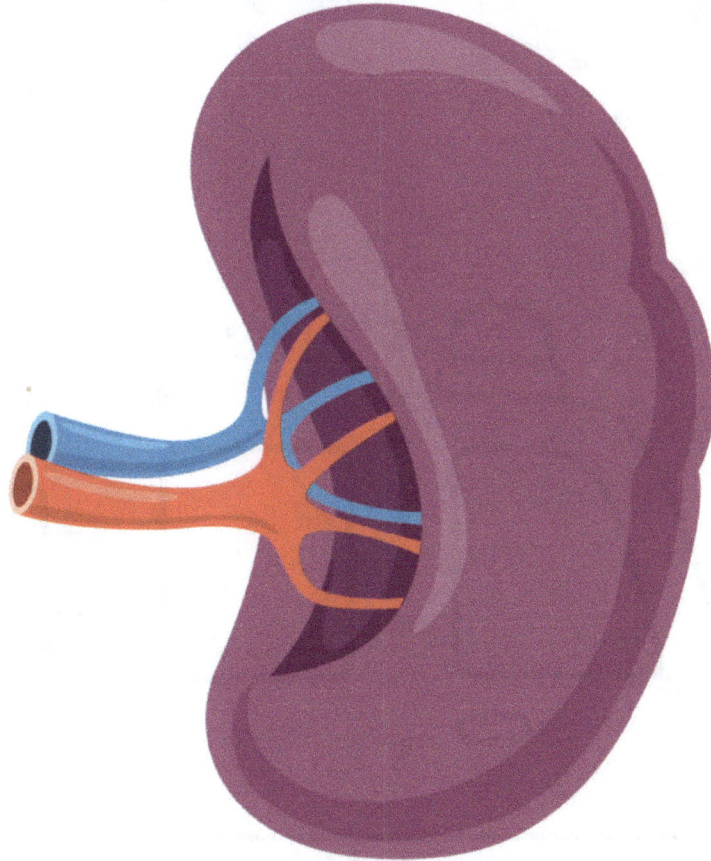

# SPLEEN

The spleen is a fist-sized organ in the upper left part of the belly under the ribcage. It helps protect the body by clearing worn-out red blood cells and germs from the bloodstream.

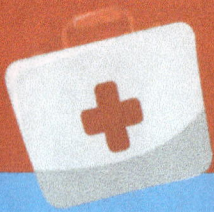

# CONNECTING DOTS

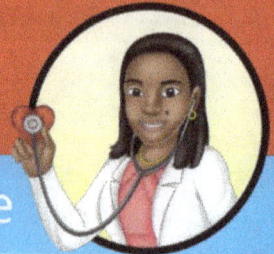

Connect the dots and color the picture

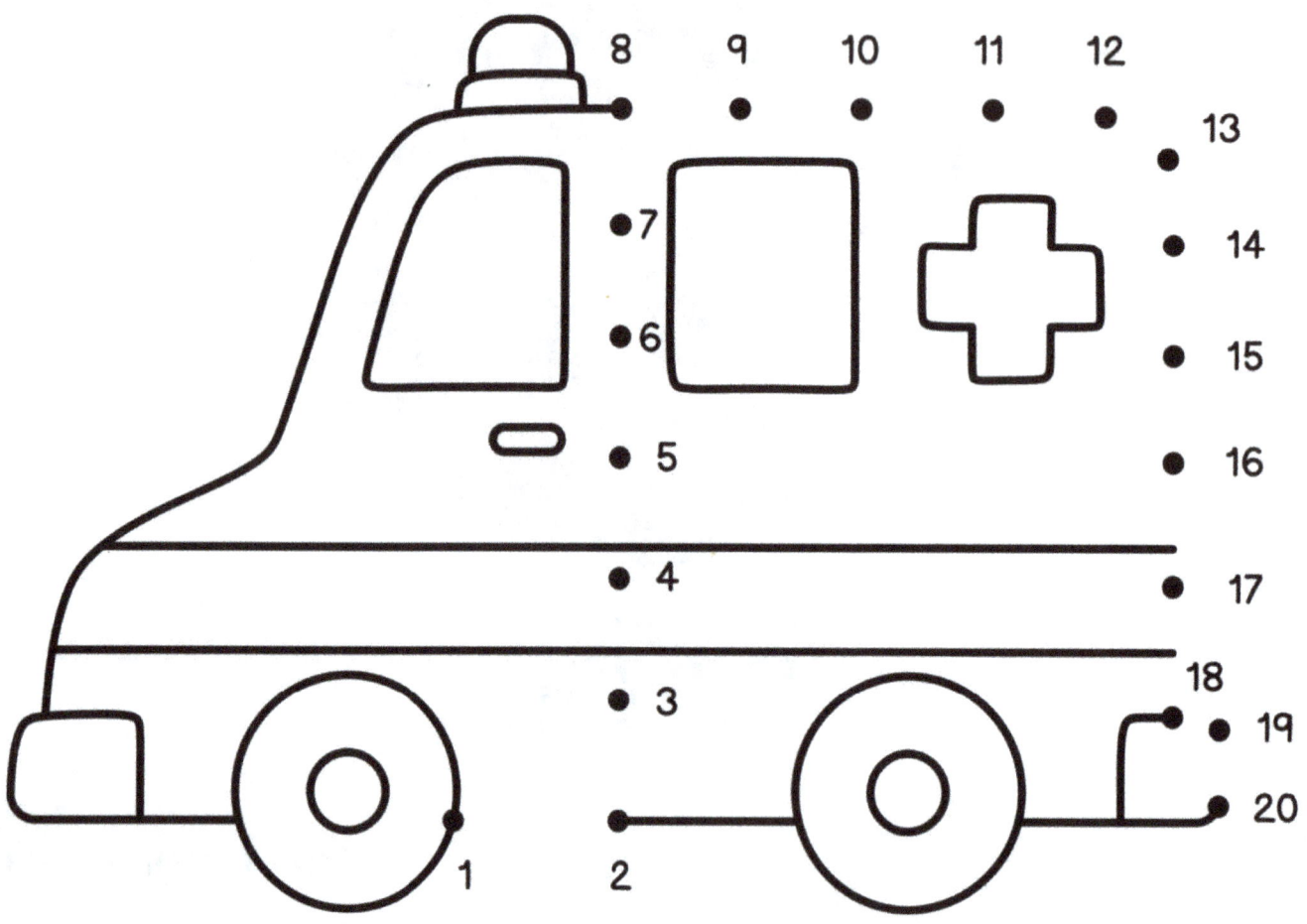

8  9  10  11  12

13

•7

14

•6

15

• 5

16

• 4

17

18

• 3

19

1   2

20

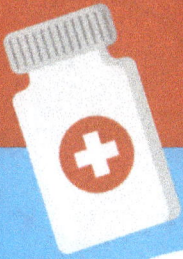
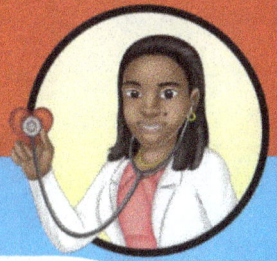

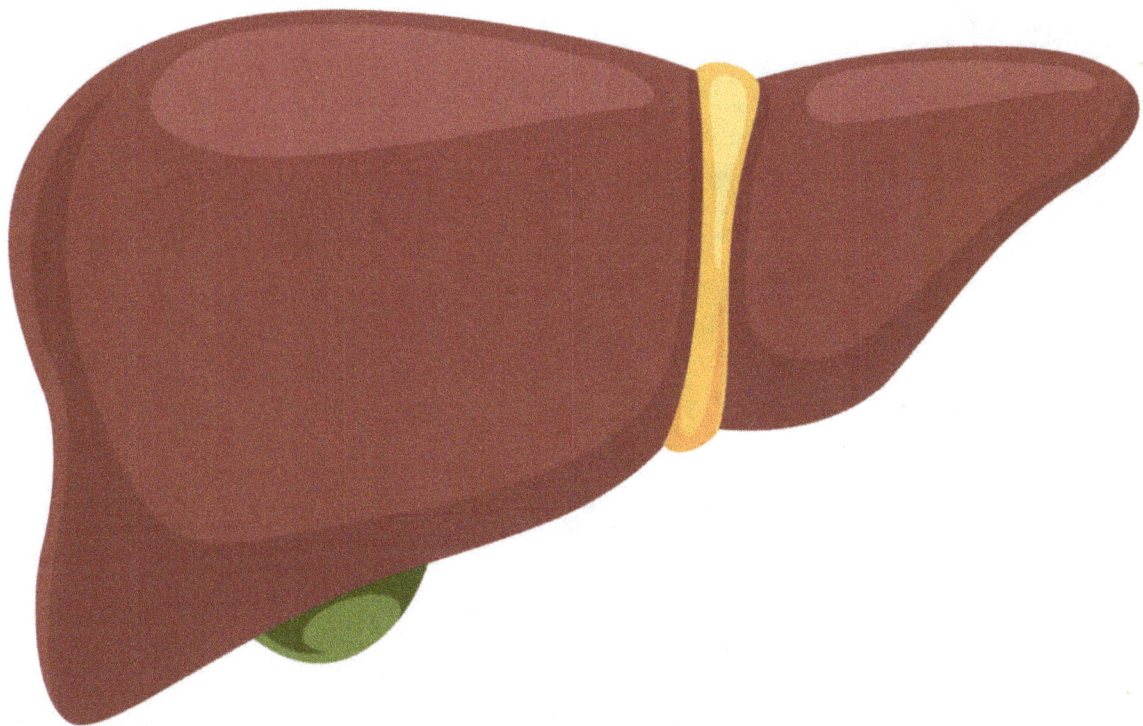

# LIVER

Your liver is the largest solid organ in your body. By the time you're grown up, it will be about the size of a football. The liver cleans your blood.

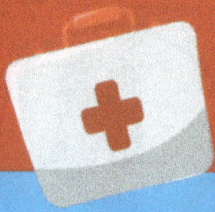

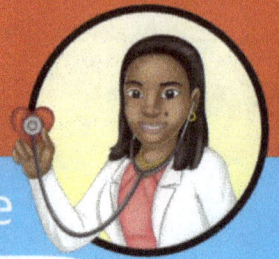

Connect the dots and color the picture

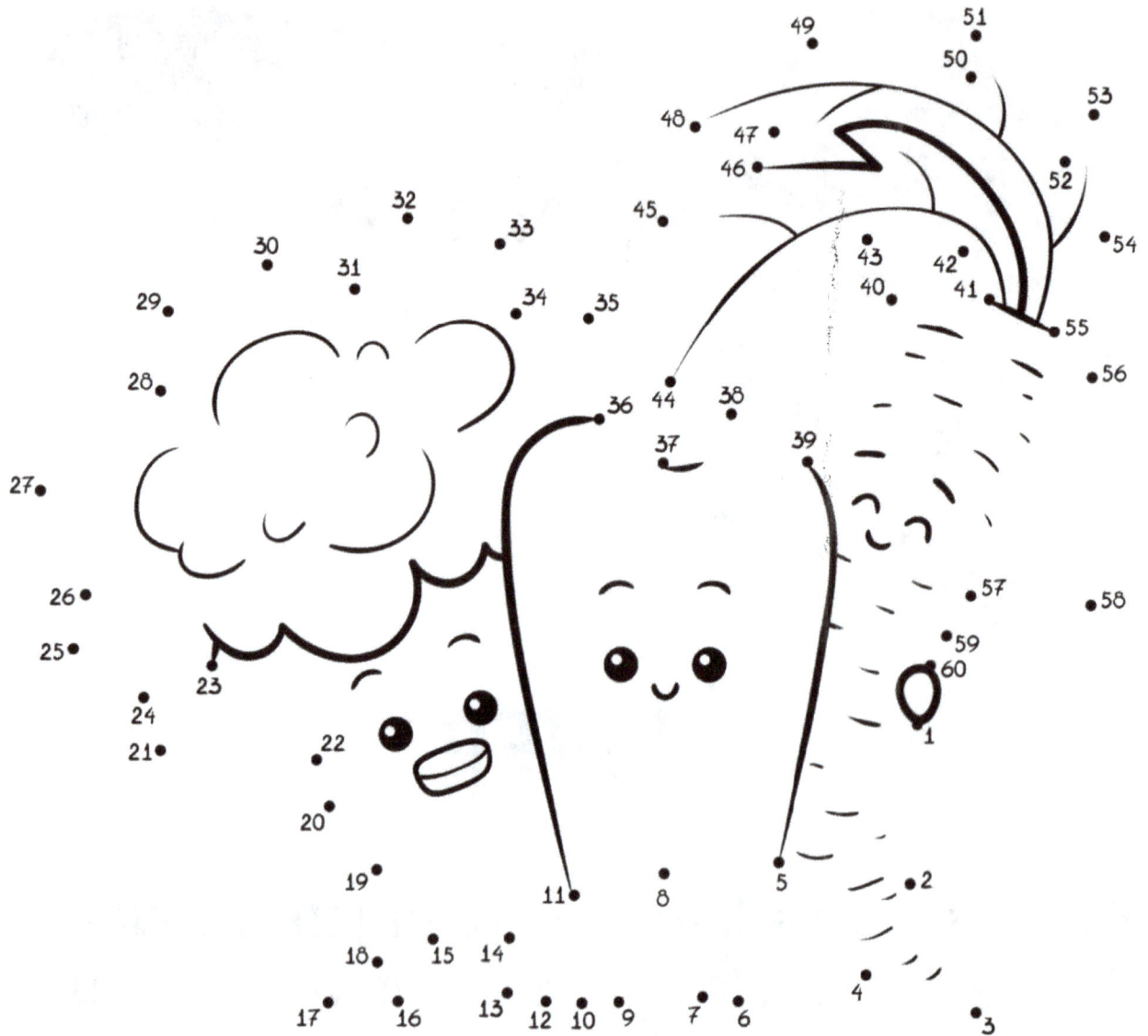

49
51
50
53
48
47
46
52
32
33
45
54
30
31
43 42
29
34 35
40 41
55
28
44 38
36 37
56
39
27
26
57
58
25
59
23
60
24
22
1
21
20
19
11 8 5 2
18 15 14
17 16 13 12 10 9 7 6
4
3

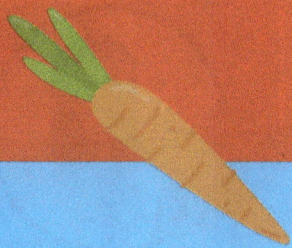

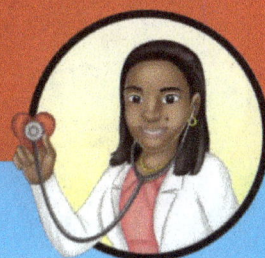

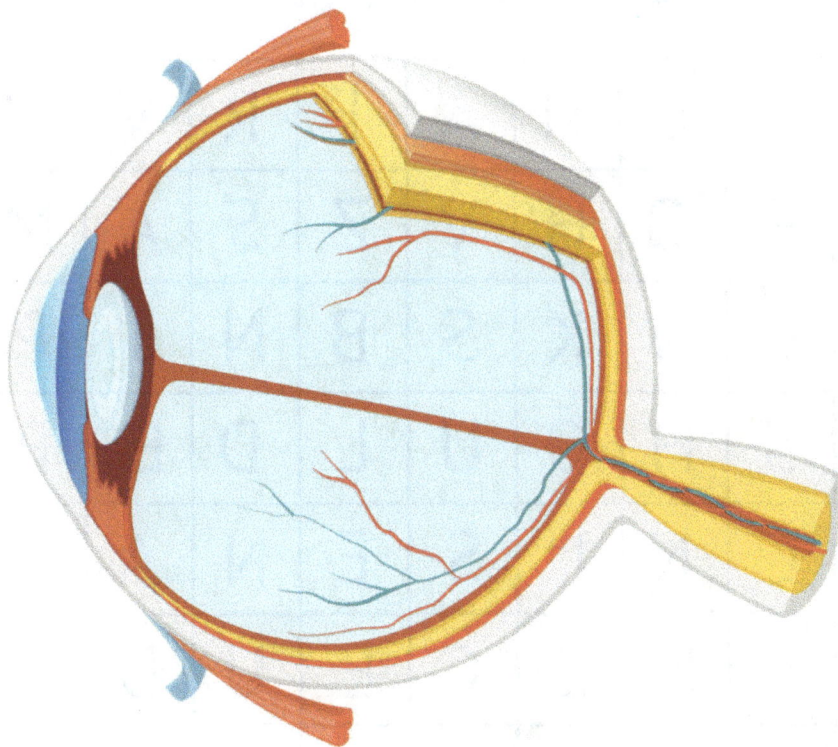

# EYE

Humans use their eyes to see.
We use our eyes from the moment we wake up
to the moment we go to sleep. They send
information to our brain. Eat plenty of carrots
to keep your eyes healthy.

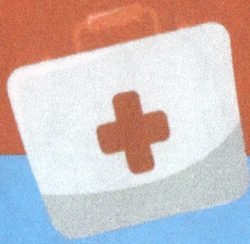

# WORD SEARCH

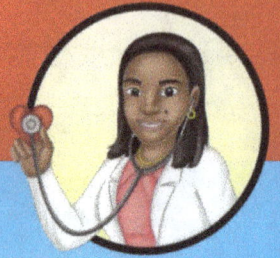

Find the hidden words

| E | D | L | H | A | I | R | V | N | E |
|---|---|---|---|---|---|---|---|---|---|
| Y | F | O | H | V | Z | S | A | M | A |
| E | G | N | K | S | B | N | J | P | R |
| B | S | H | O | U | L | D | E | R | S |
| R | C | N | L | S | E | N | A | K | E |
| O | E | M | B | C | E | U | D | Q | C |
| W | H | O | Y | G | T | B | X | K | H |
| S | J | U | Y | M | E | Y | E | S | E |
| F | A | T | O | N | G | U | E | V | E |
| D | F | H | N | E | C | K | Y | B | K |

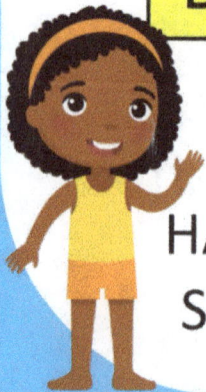

## WORDS

HAIR – EARS – CHEEK – EYEBROWS – NOSE
SHOULDERS – MOUTH – NECK – TONGUE

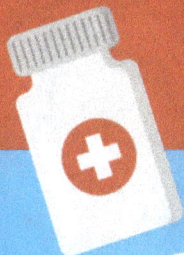
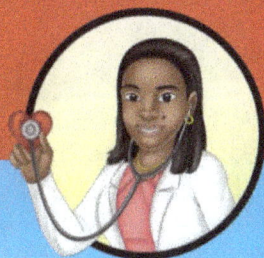

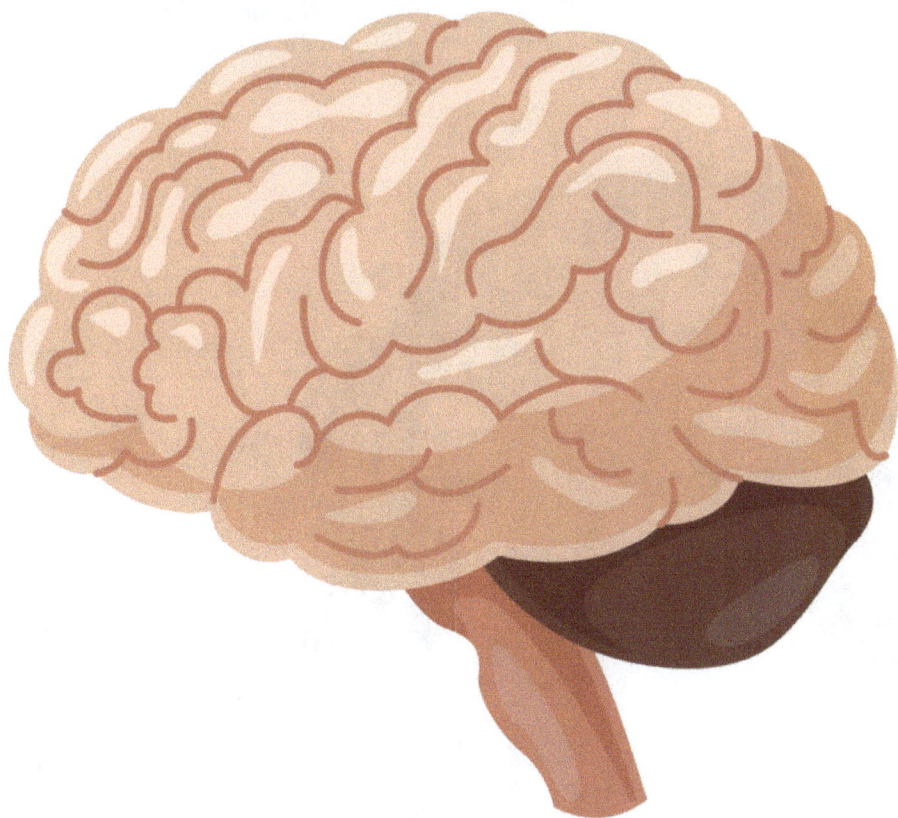

# BRAIN

The brain is the control center for the body. As a part of the nervous system, the brain receives and makes sense of signals sent from nerve cells in the body. The brain also sends information to the body's muscles and organs.

# HEALTHY FOOD

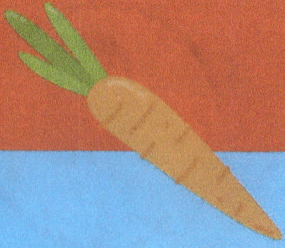

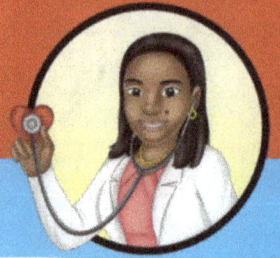

## Circle the healthy foods

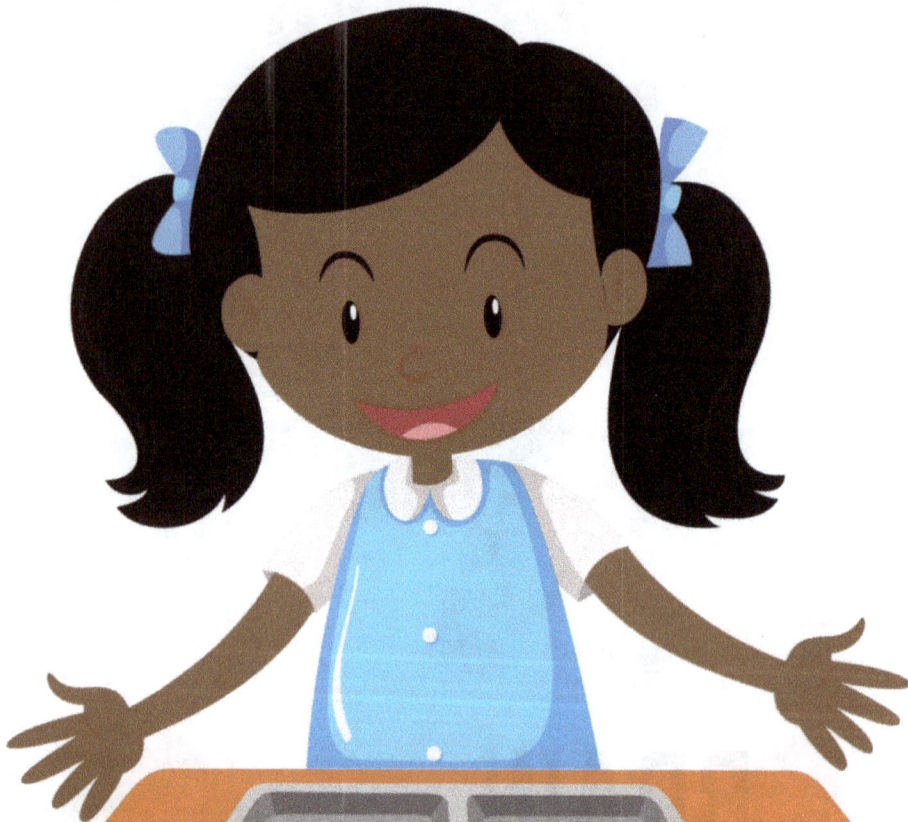

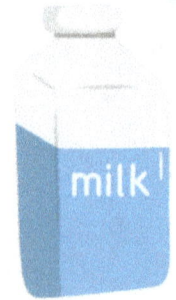

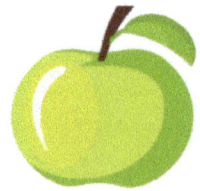

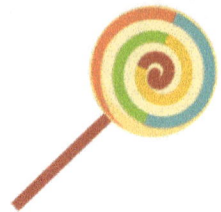

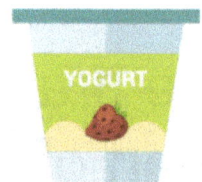

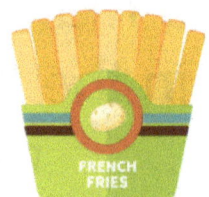

milk

YOGURT

FRENCH FRIES

# MAZE

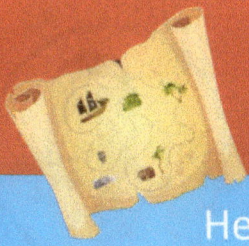

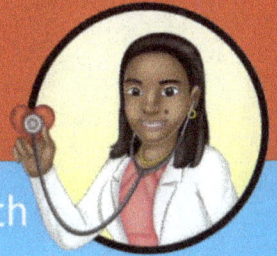

Help the toothbrush and toothpaste find the tooth

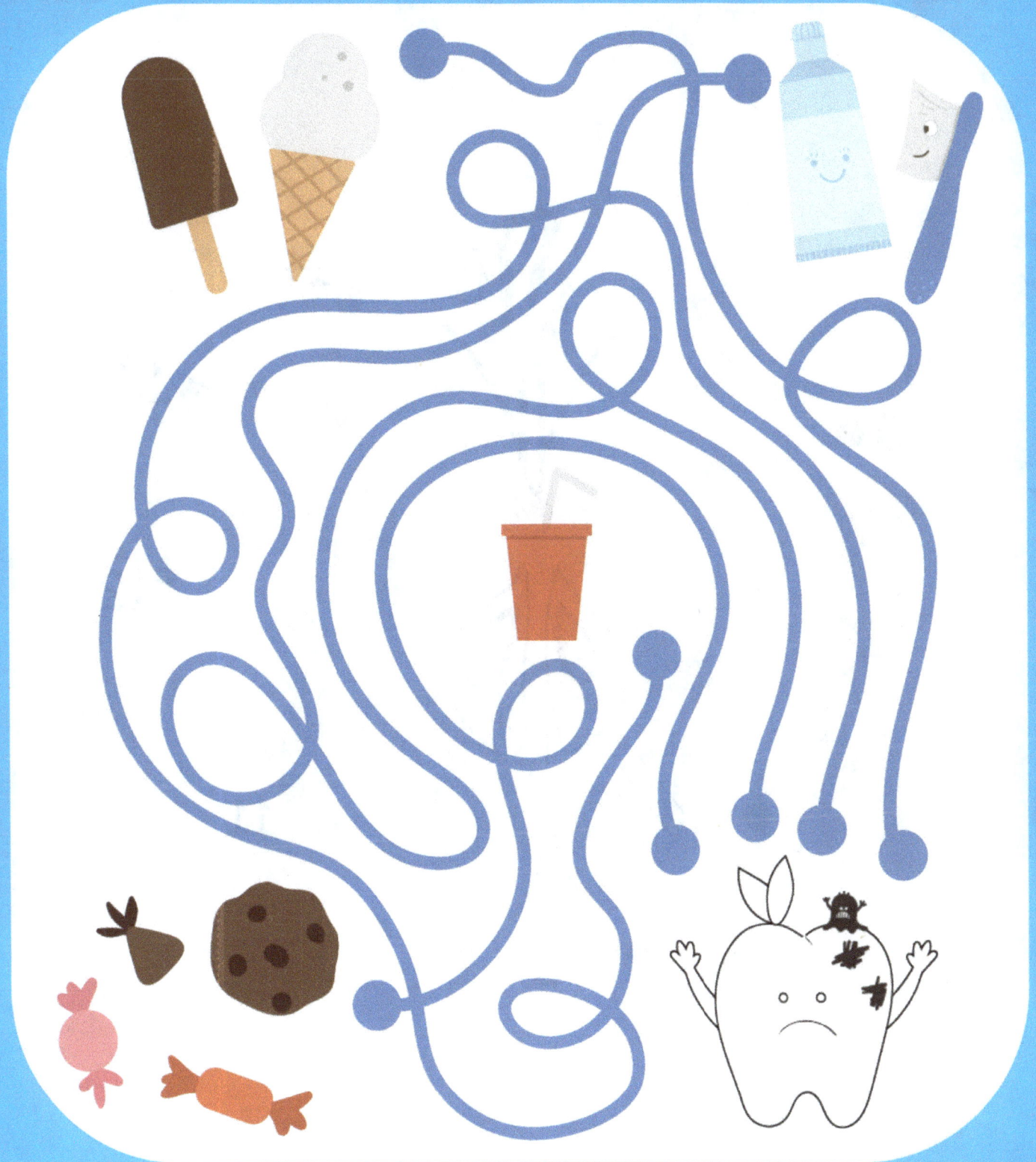

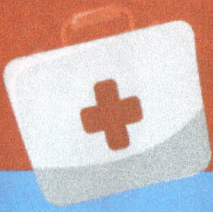

# CONNECTING DOTS

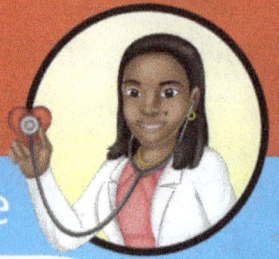

Connect the dots and color the picture

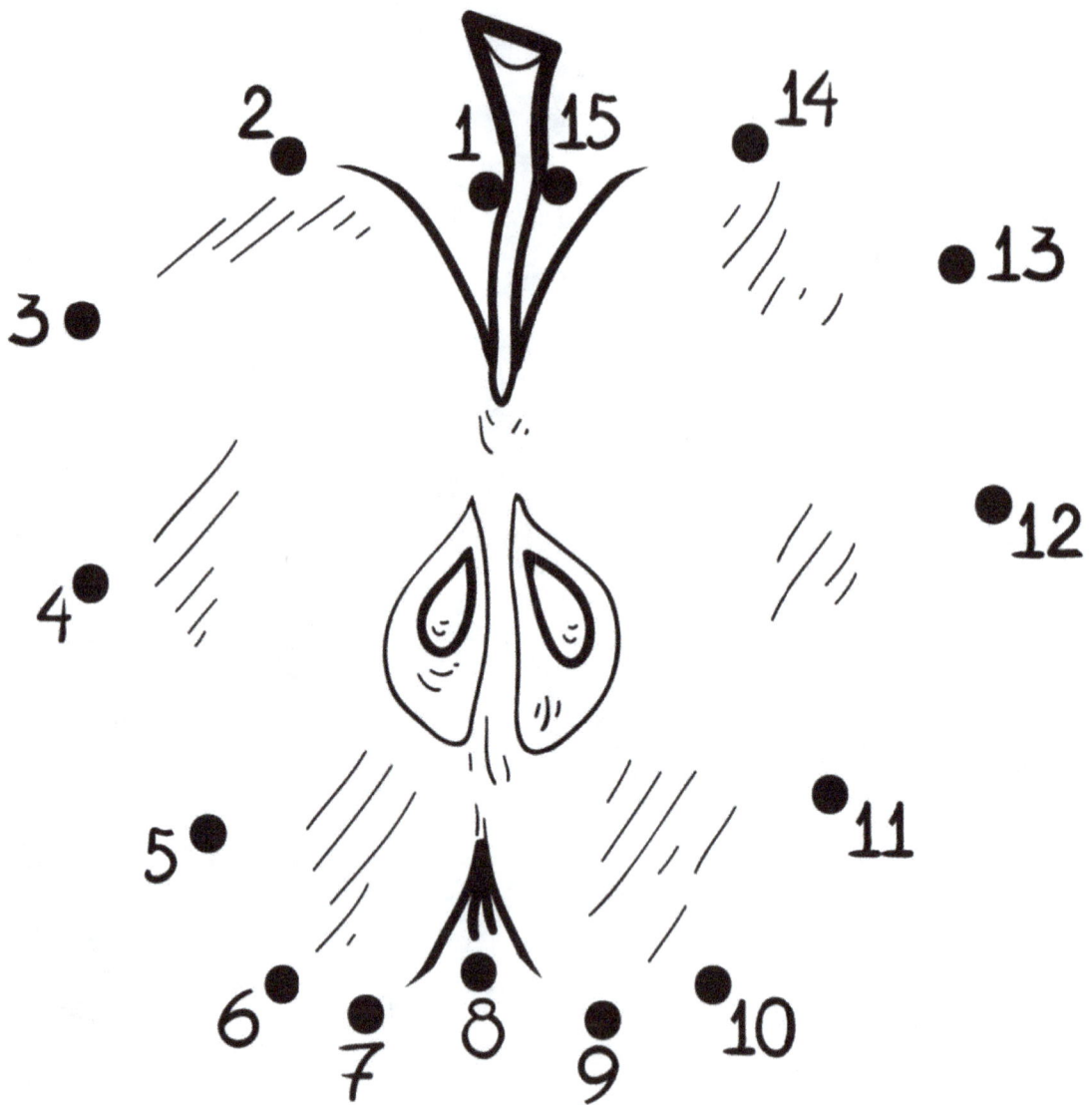

2

1  15

14

3

13

4

12

5

11

6

7  8  9  10

# MAZE

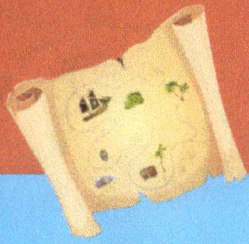

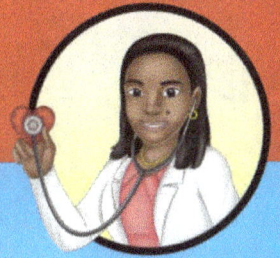

Help the tooth find the dentist

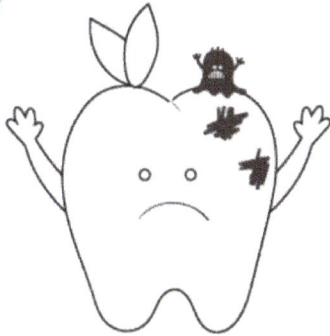

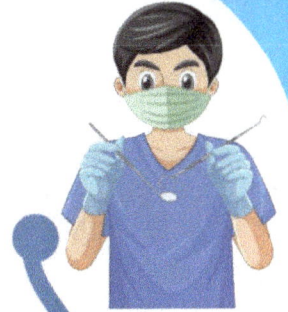

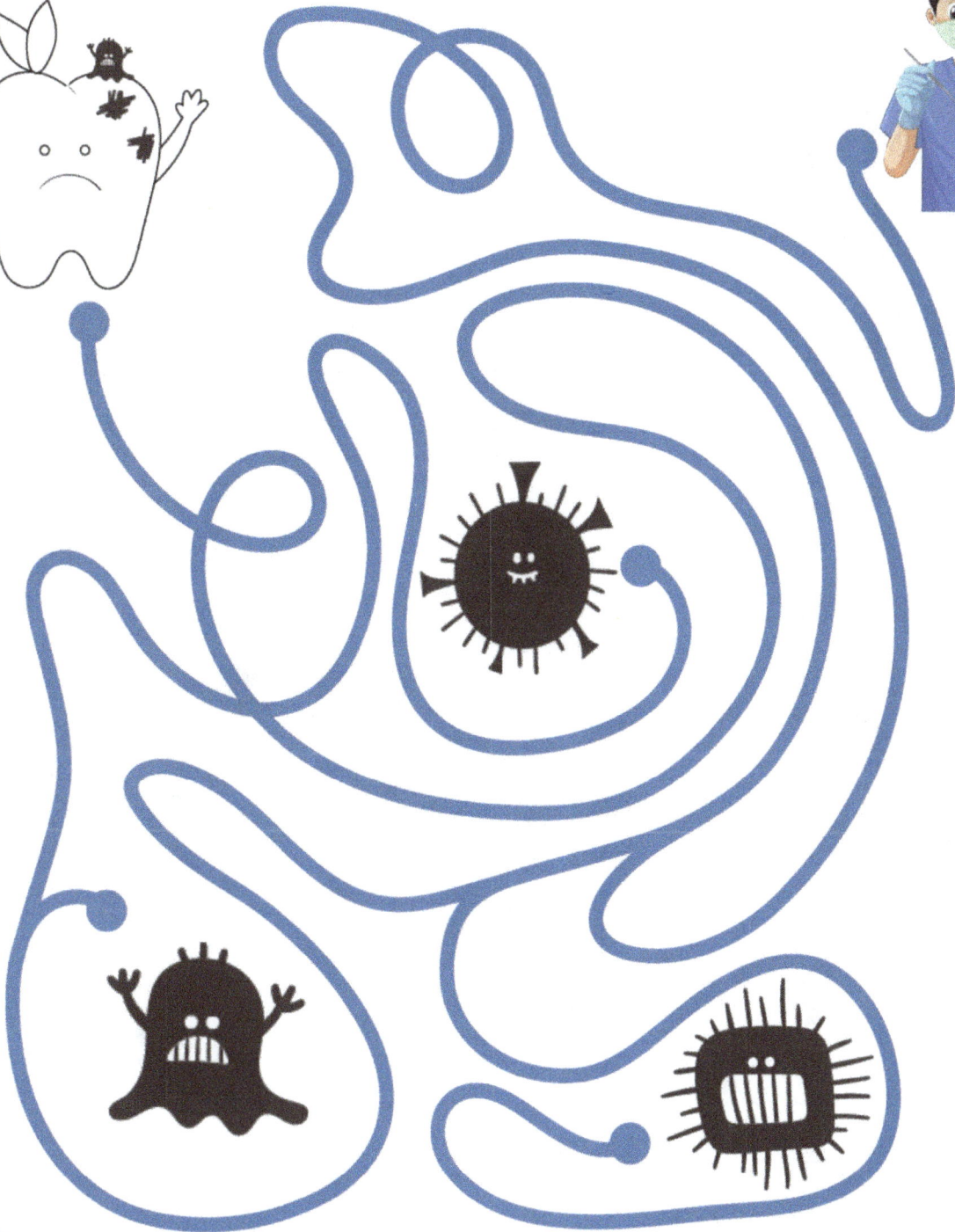

# REPRODUCTIVE SYSTEM

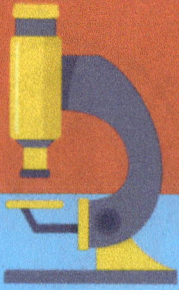

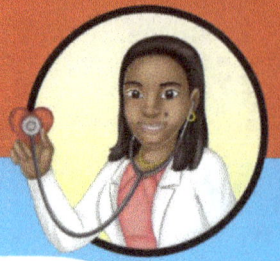

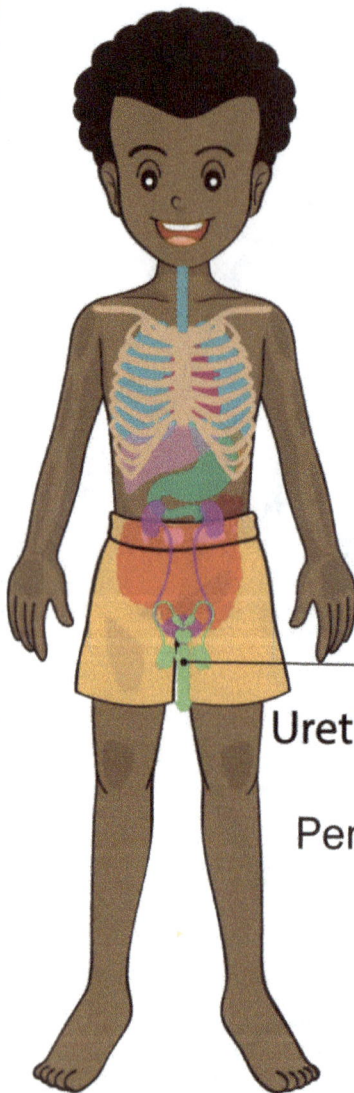

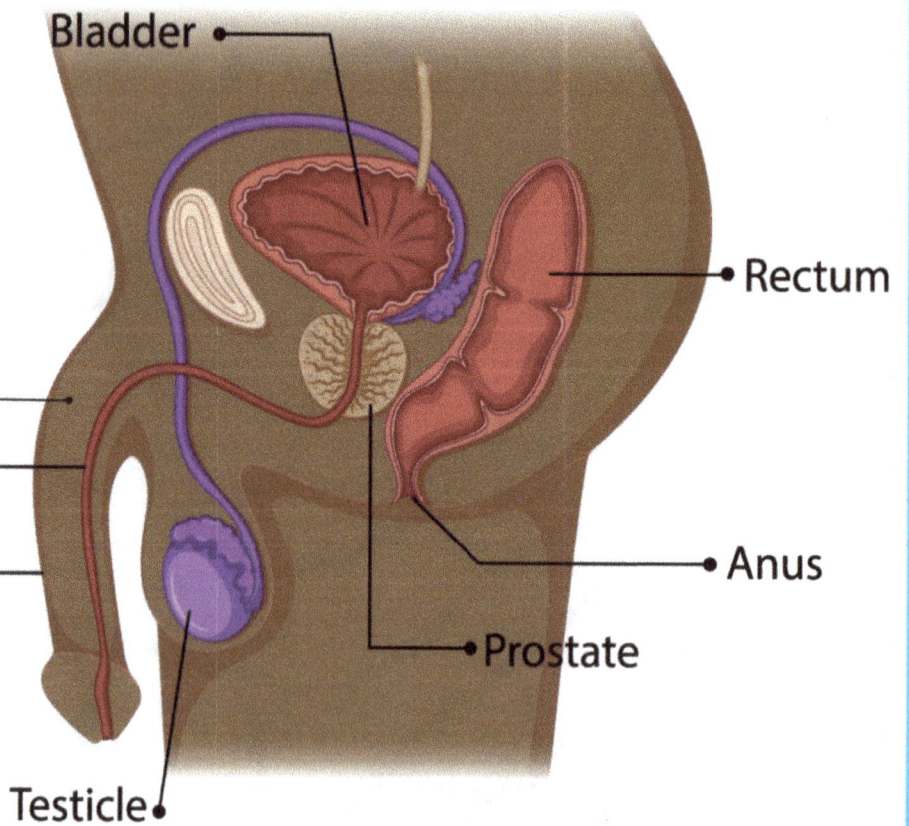

Bladder

Rectum

Urethra

Penis

Anus

Prostate

Testicle

# REPRODUCTIVE SYSTEM

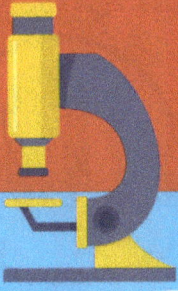

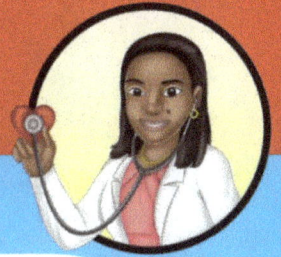

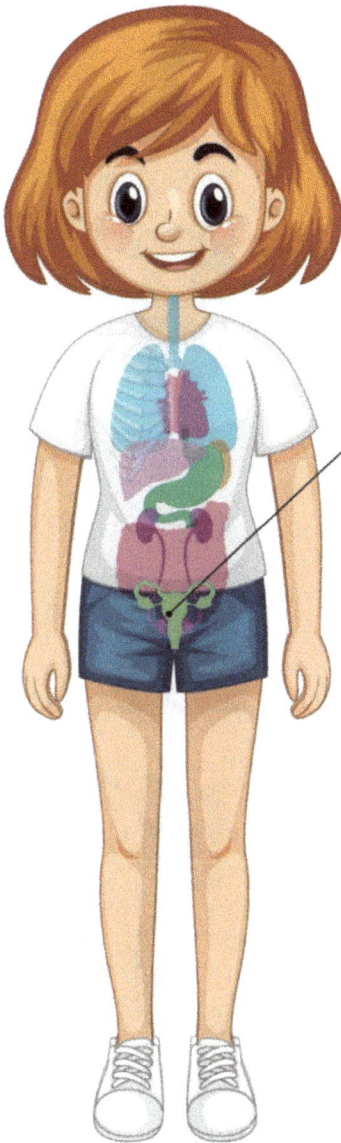

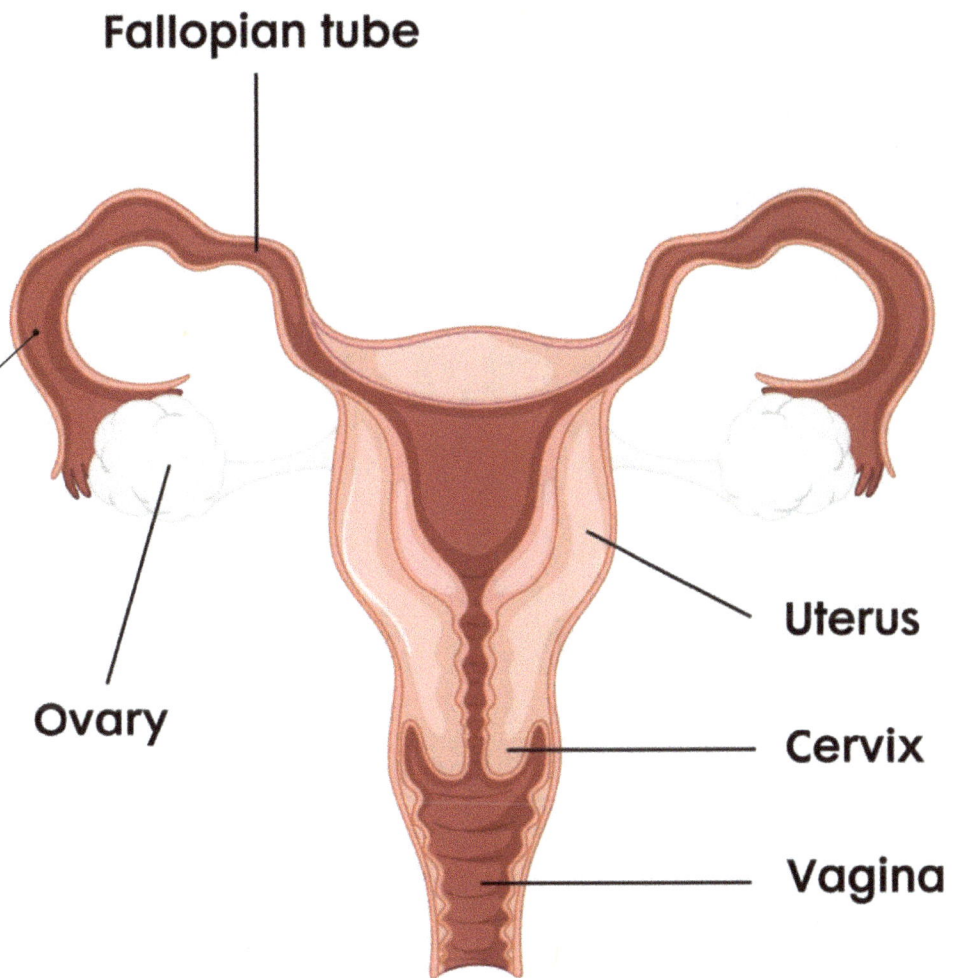

Fallopian tube

Ovary

Uterus

Cervix

Vagina

# MATCHING

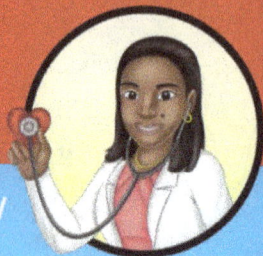

Match each picture with the correct shadow

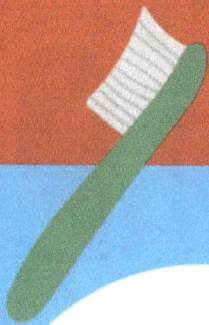

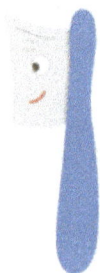

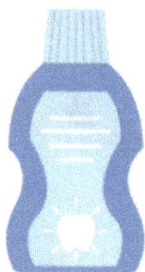

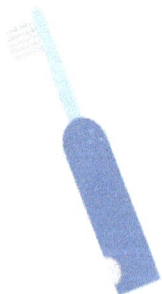

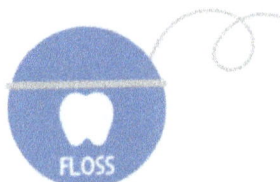

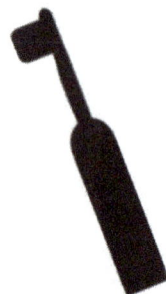

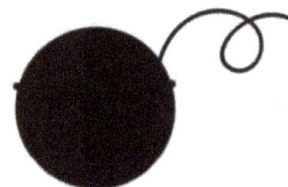

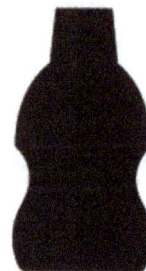

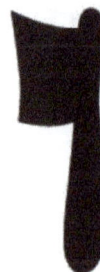

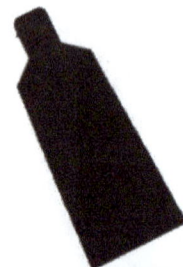

# COLORING TIME!

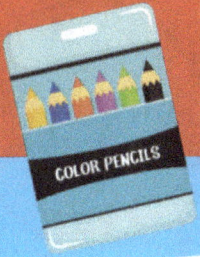

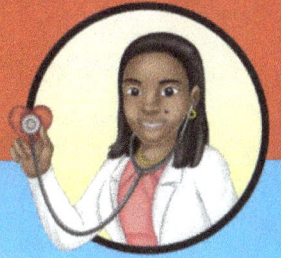

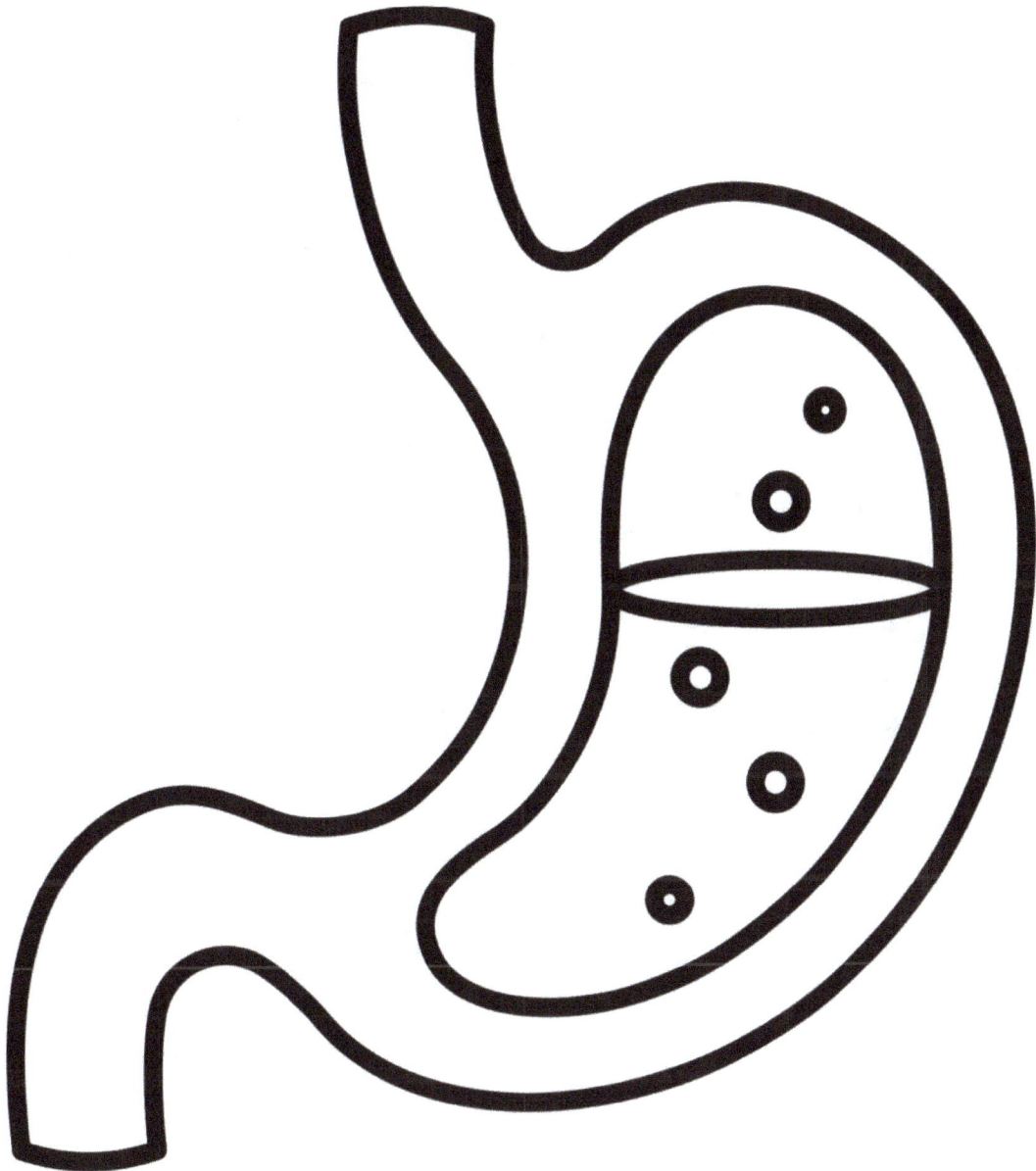

STOMACH

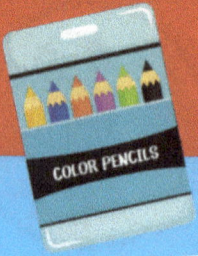
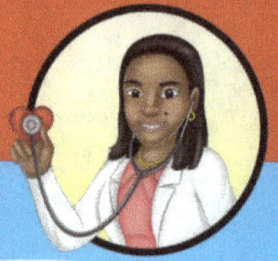

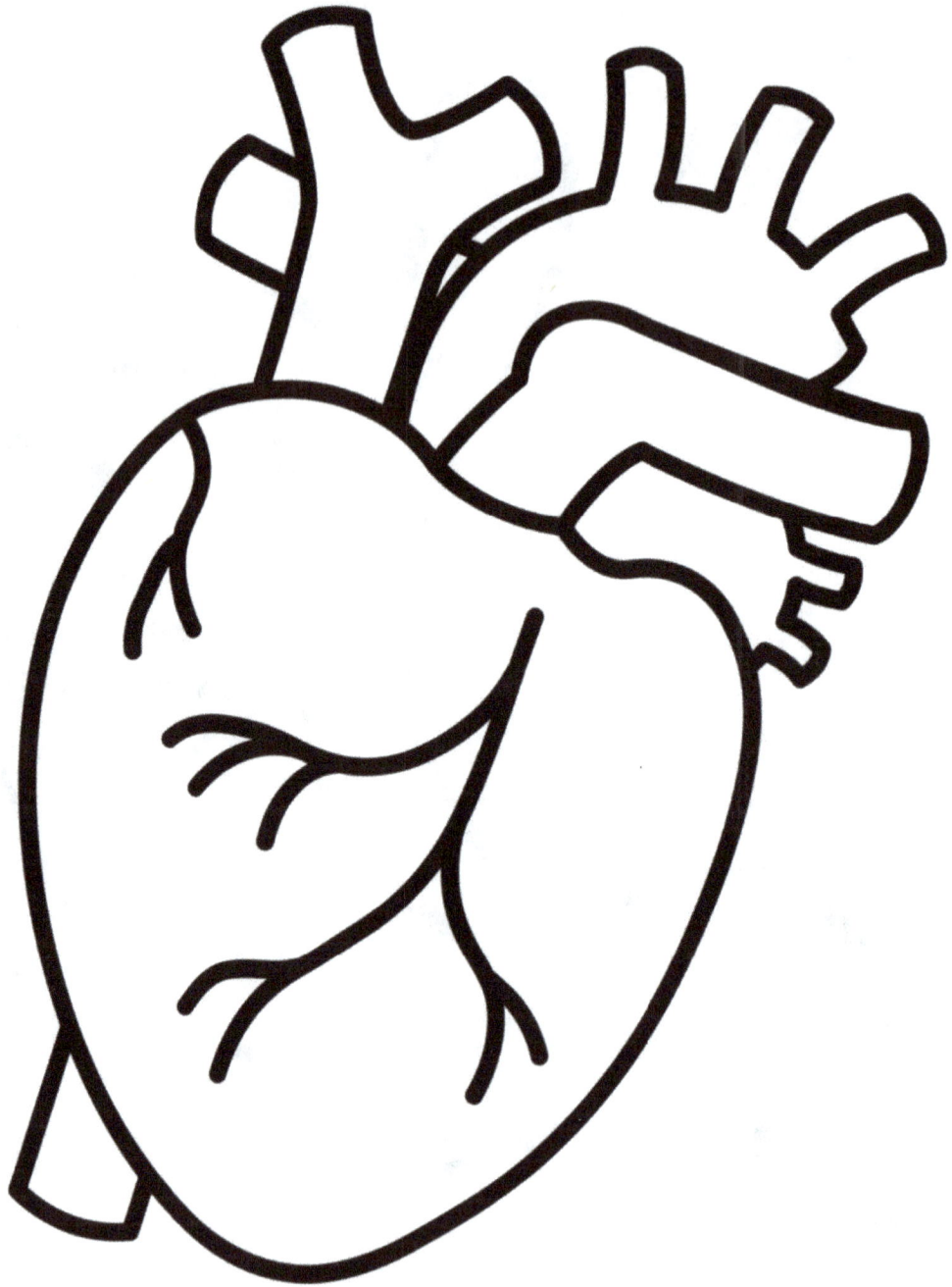

# HEART

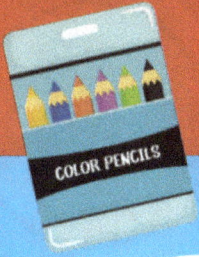

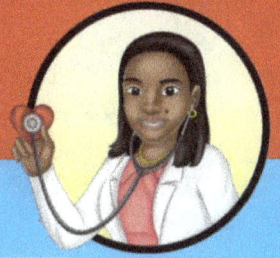

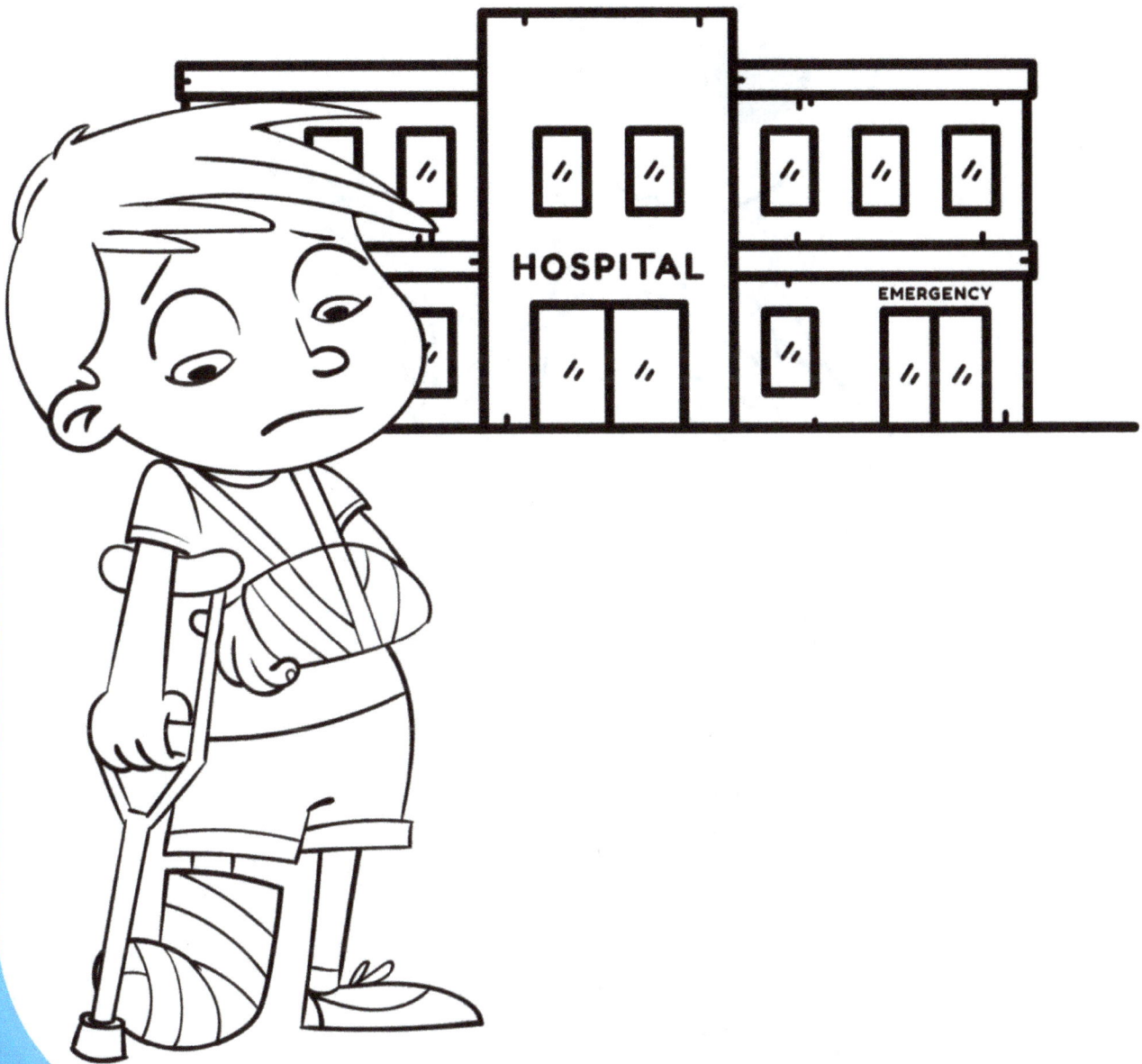

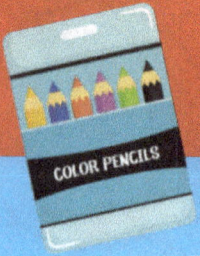

# COLORING TIME!

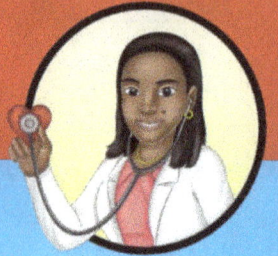

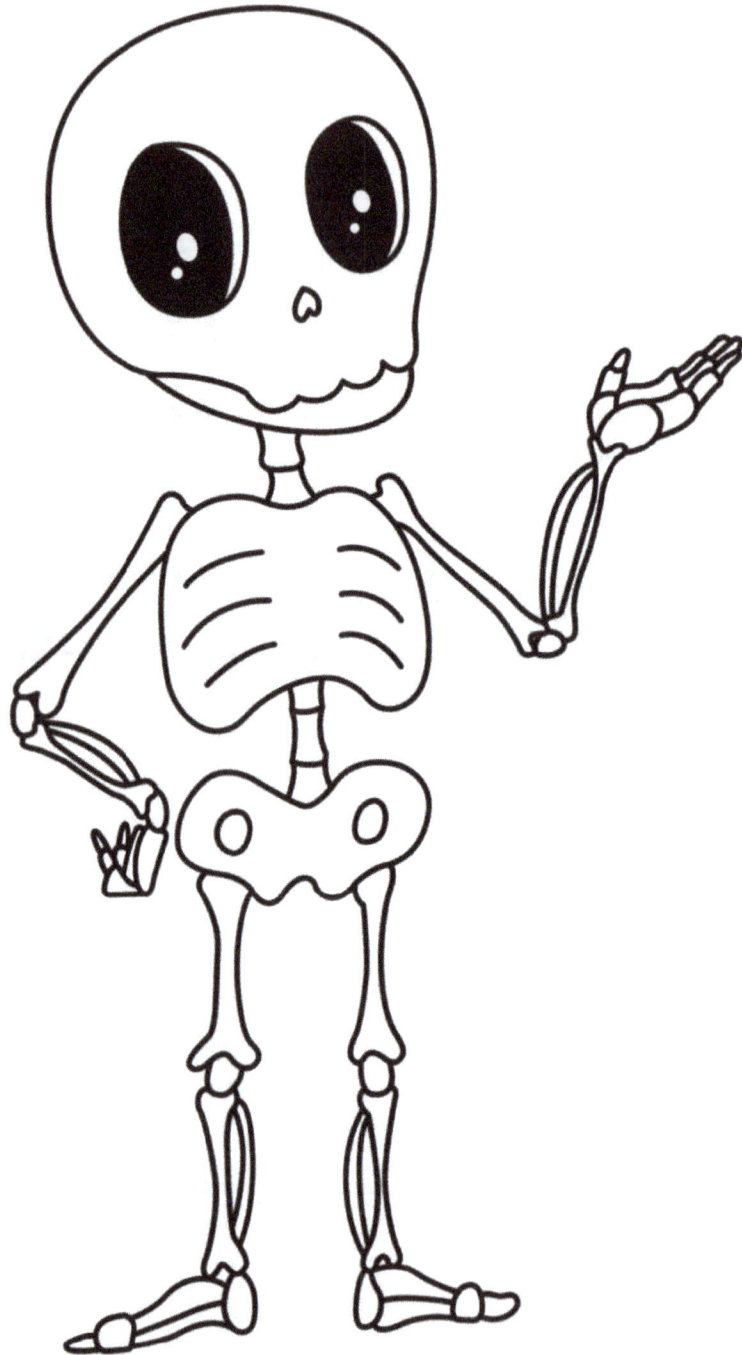

# COLORING TIME!

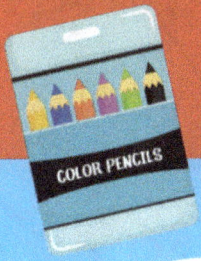

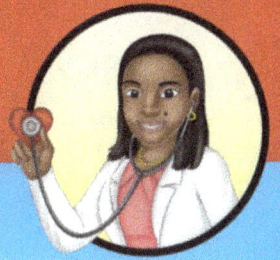

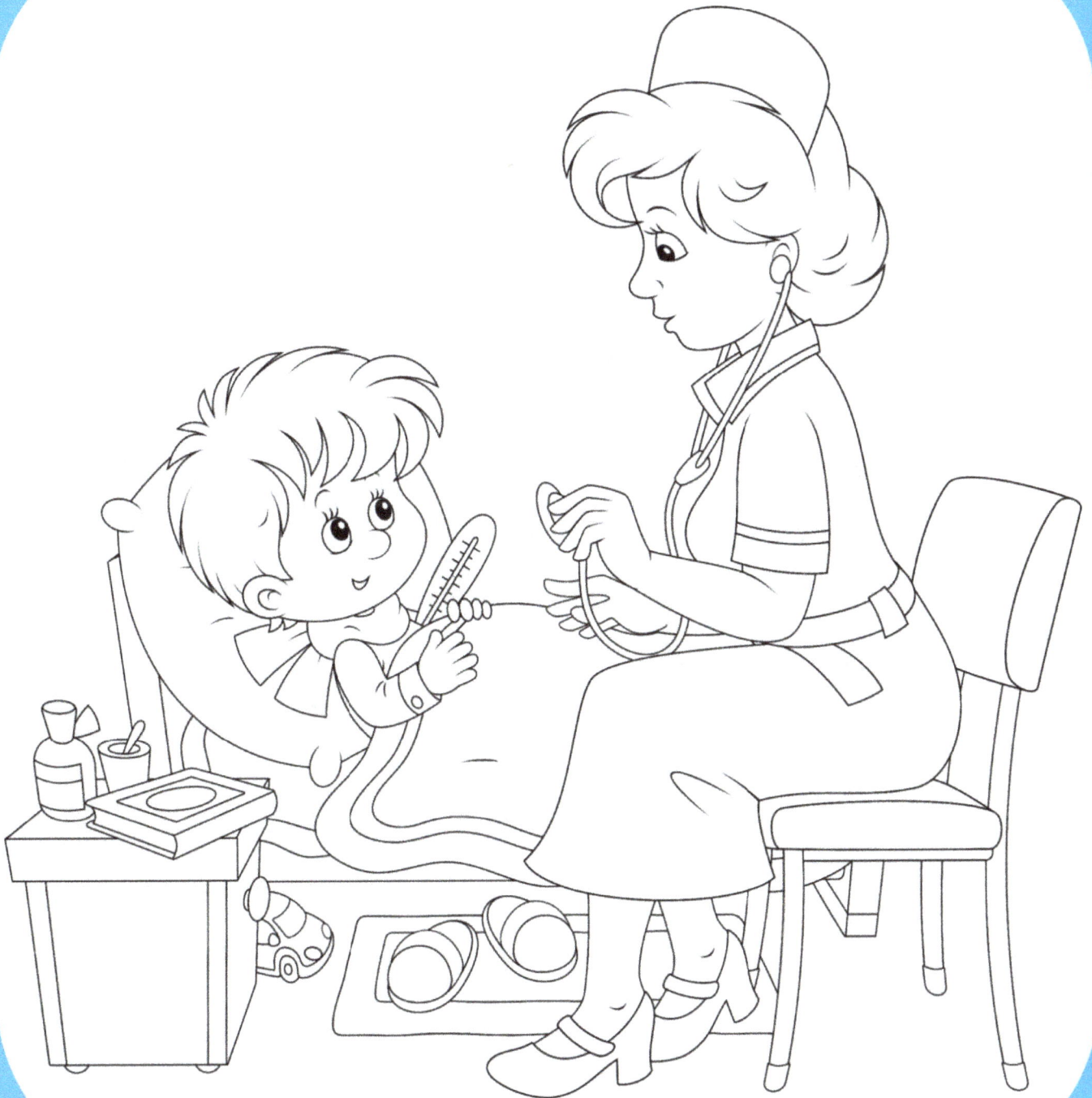

# COLORING TIME!

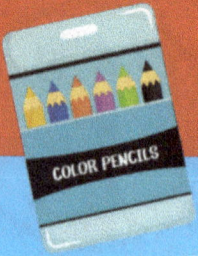

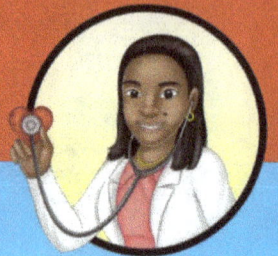

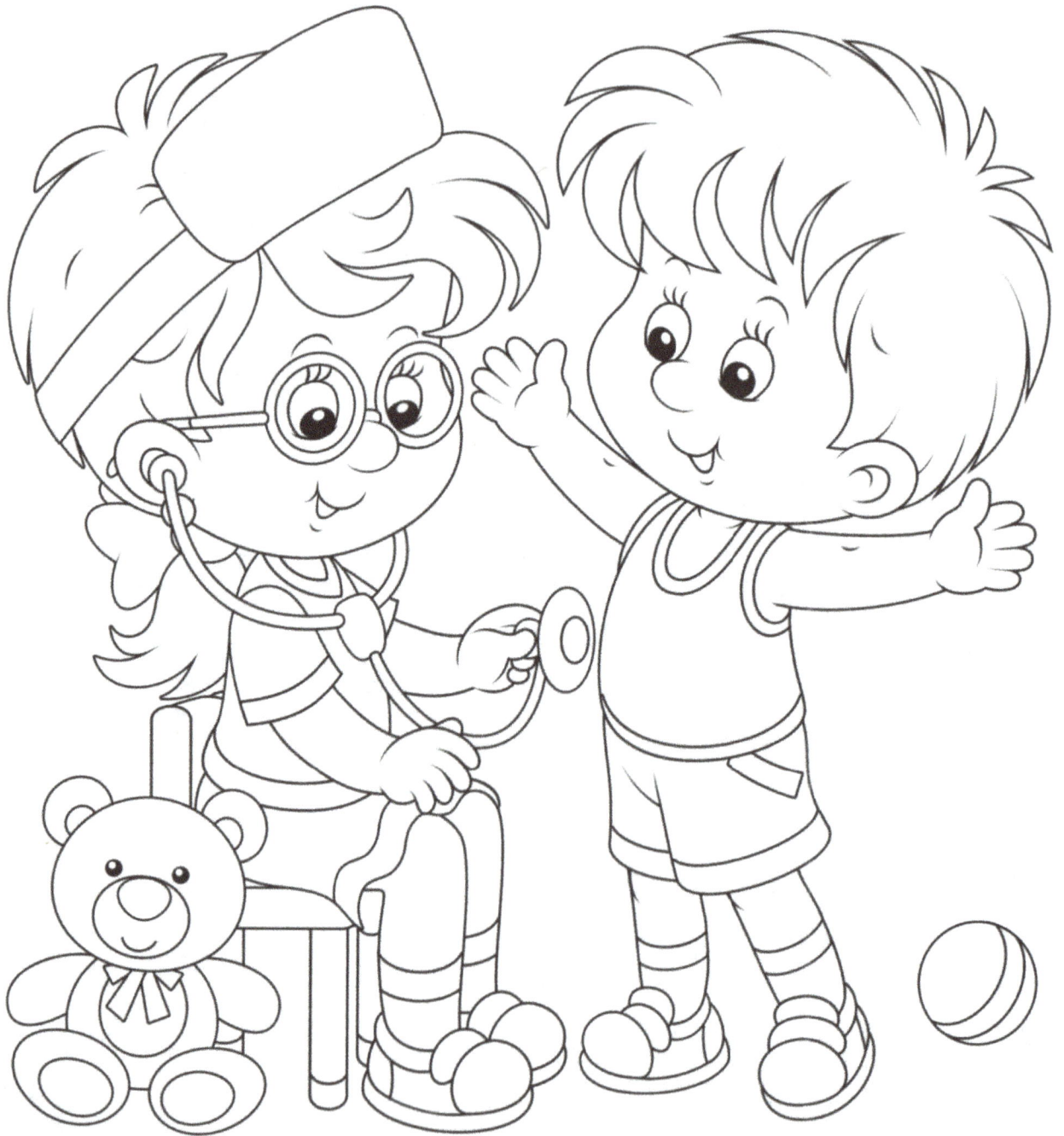

COLOR PENCILS

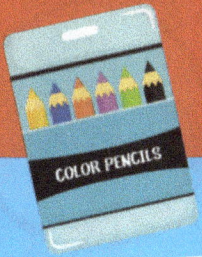

# COLORING TIME!

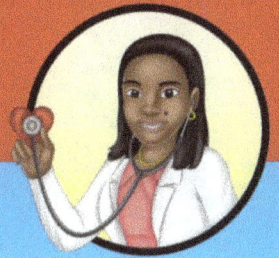

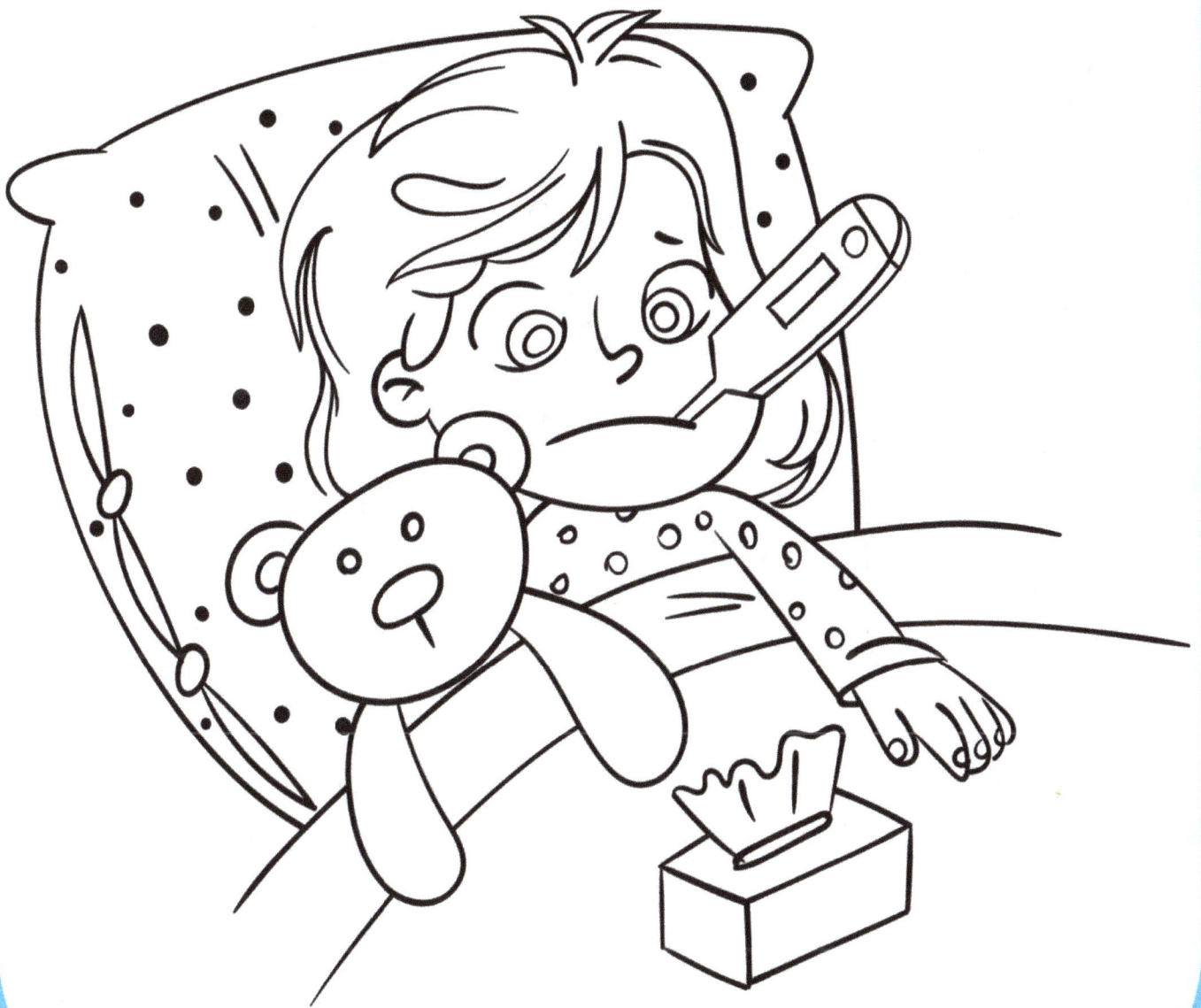

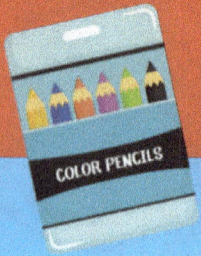
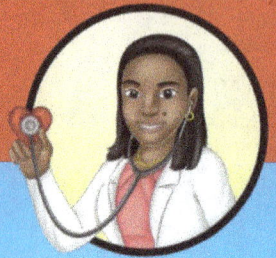
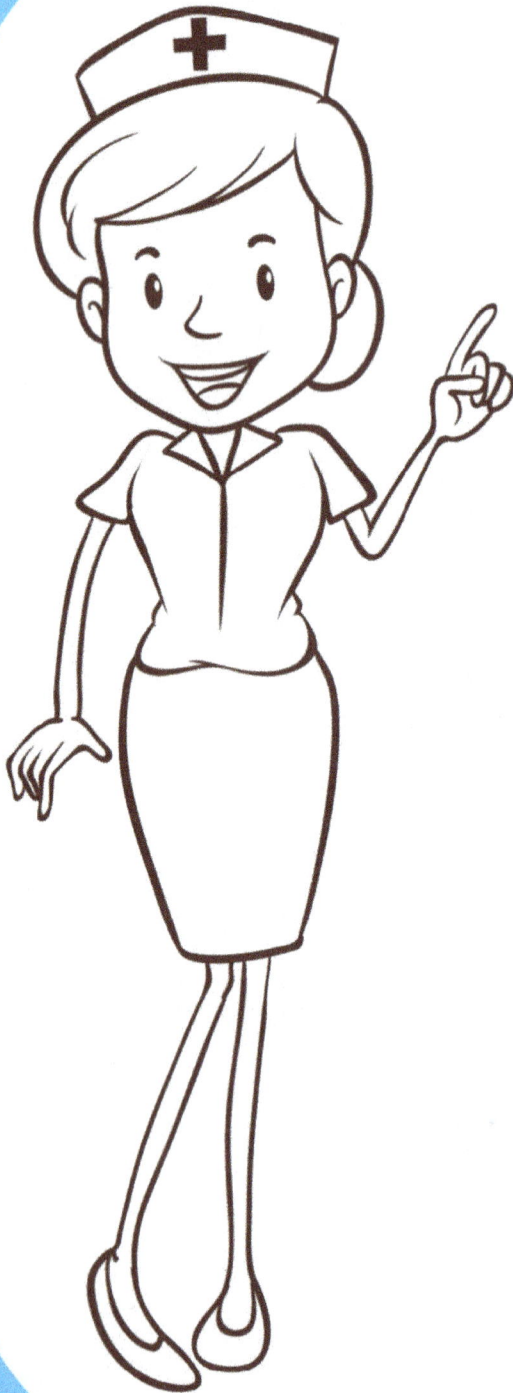
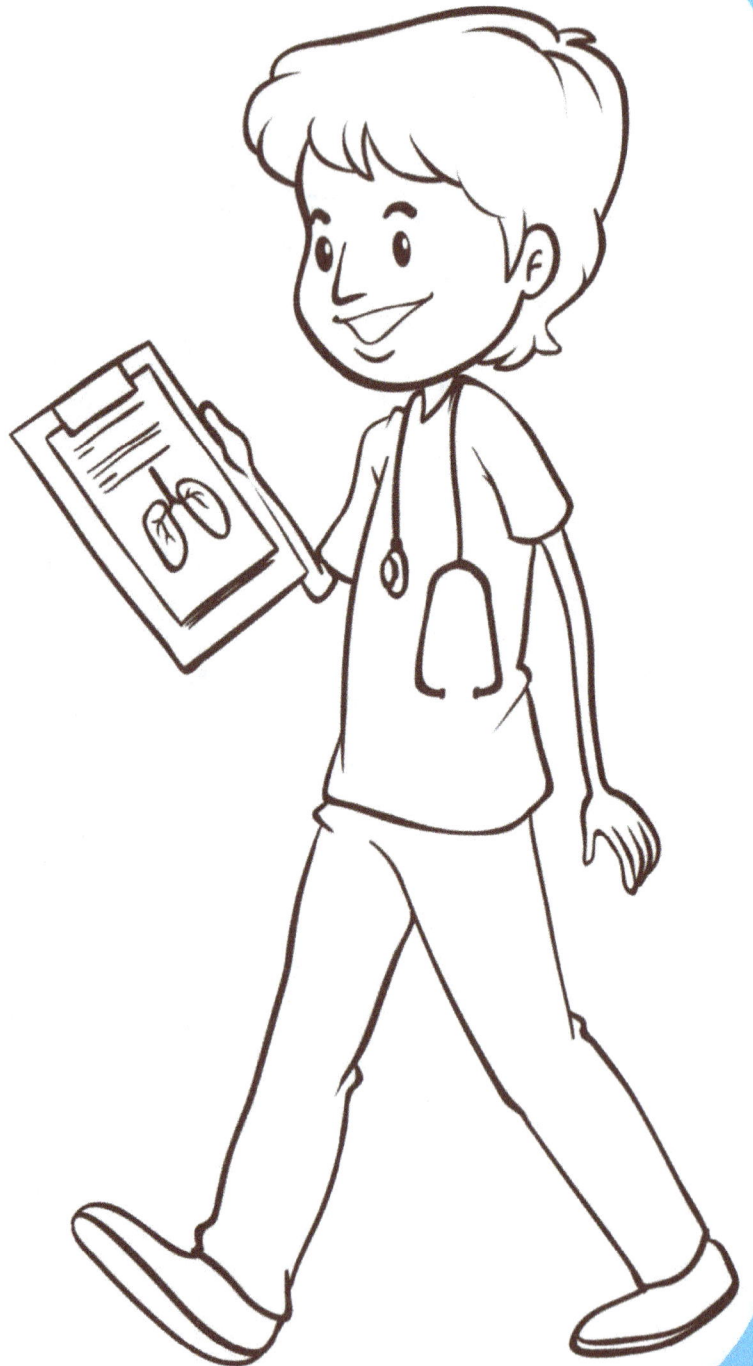

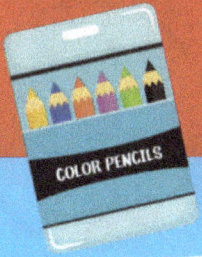

we love to exercise

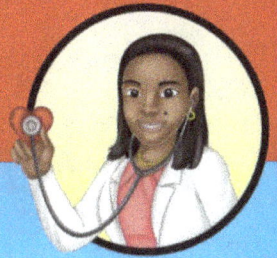

## COLOR THE PICTURE

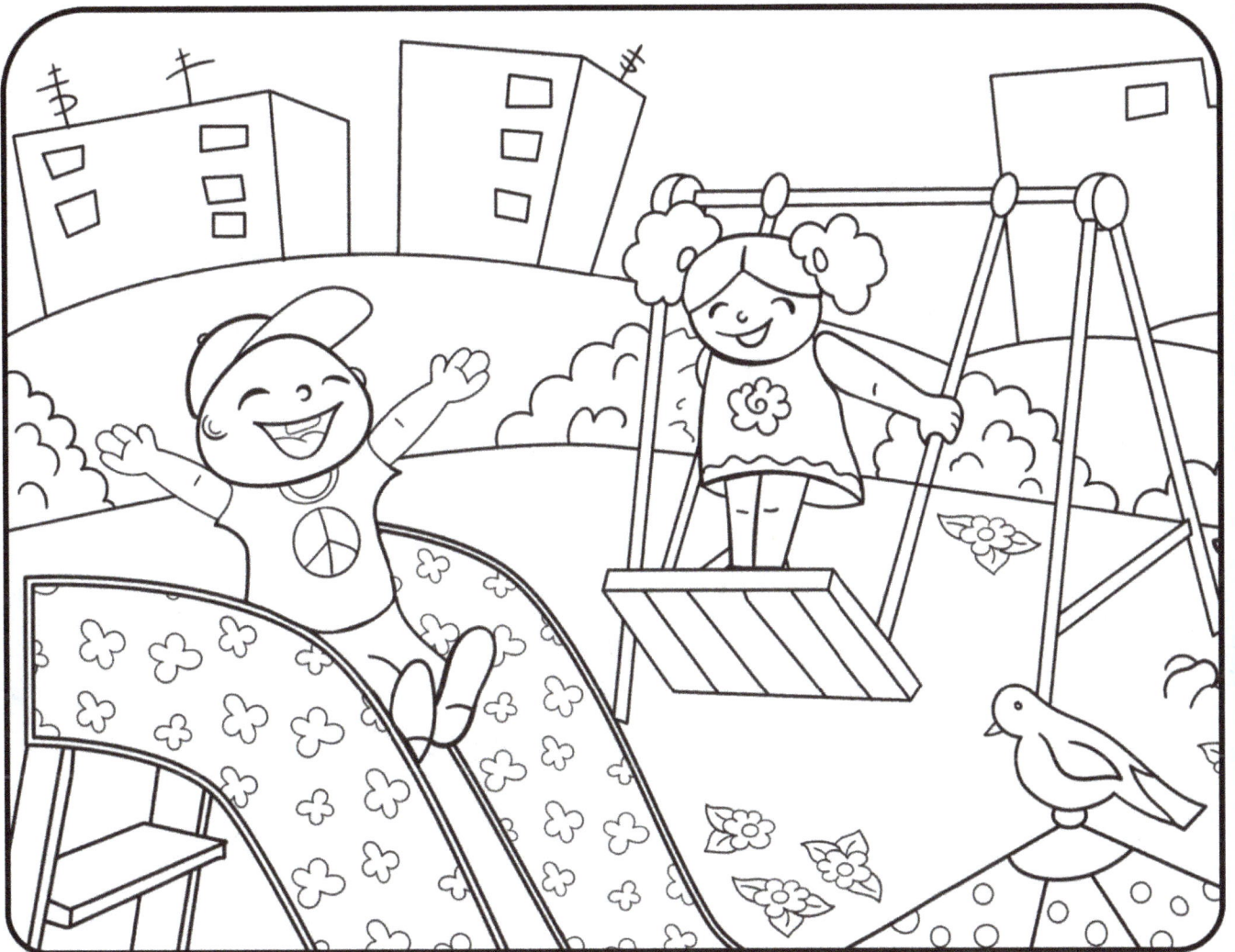

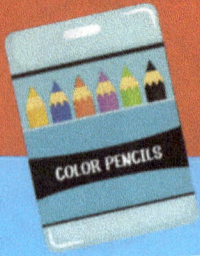

# COLORING TIME!

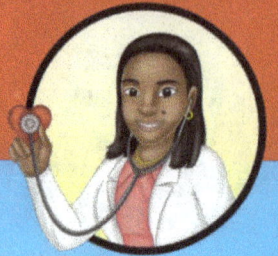

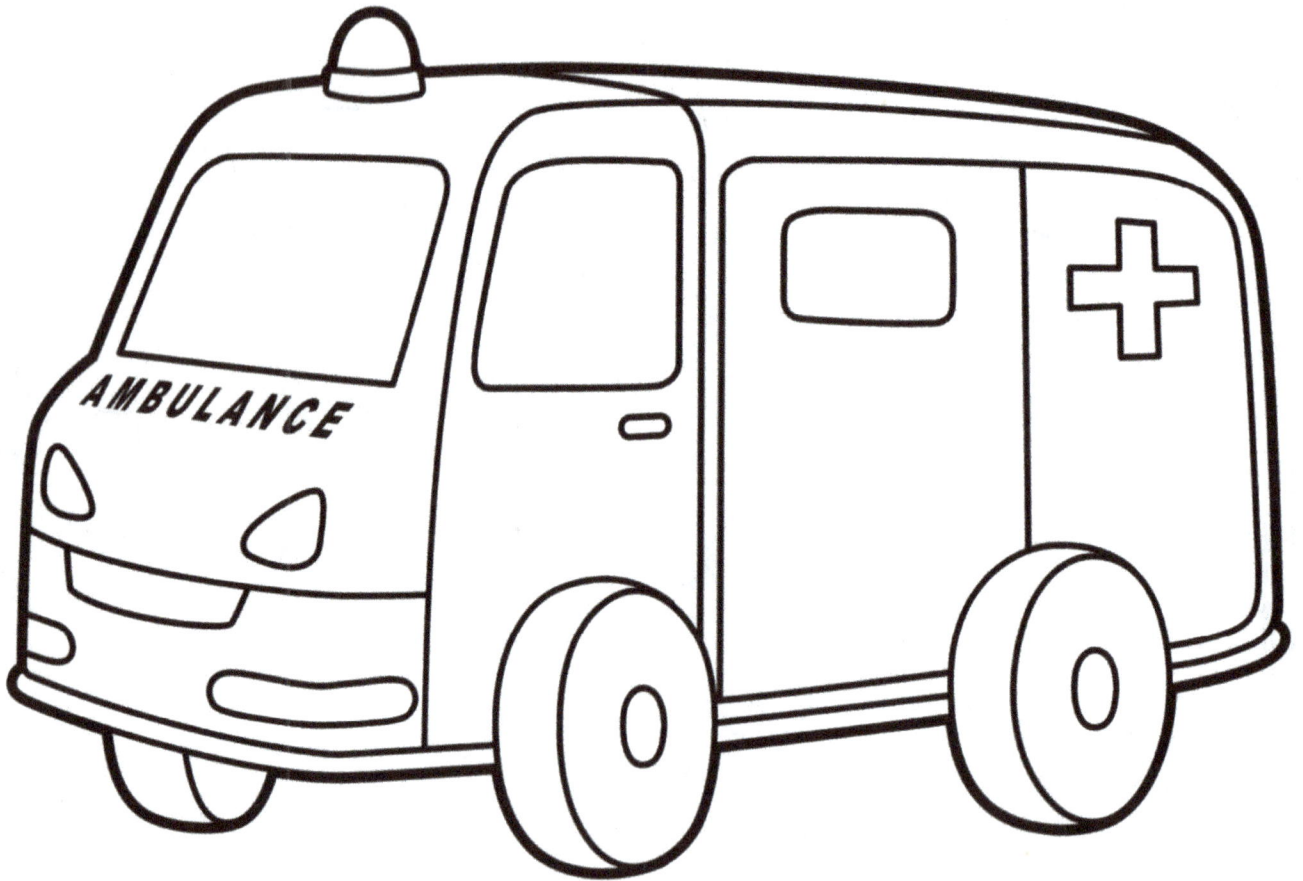

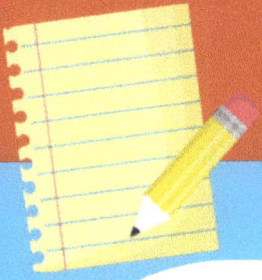

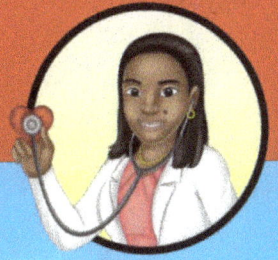

# FUN FACTS TO REMEMBER

1. There are 32 permanent teeth in the human mouth.

2. Normal body temperature is generally 98.6 °F (37 °C).

3. The adult human skeleton consists of about 206 bones.

4. The human brain is 80% water.

5. It takes 17 muscles to smile and about 48 muscles to frown.

☺ KEEP SMILING!

www.ingramcontent.com/pod-product-compliance
Lightning Source LLC
Chambersburg PA
CBHW080427030426
42335CB00020B/2617